The Truth About CBD - Using Cannabidiol as a Medication – Case Studies and Real Life Stories Revealed

By:

Ray Tokes

Over the last five years, a slow revolution has been sweeping quietly across the globe.

Public attitudes towards both the medicinal and recreational use of marijuana are changing. [1] Now, an increasing number of countries are deciding to either legalize the drug or relax laws governing its use. [2] As this cultural shift has just as many critics as it does champions, the future of marijuana use in America, the UK, South America, and Europe remains certain.

However, these developments are already having an impact on the accessibility and application of CBD.

CBD currently occupies a bit of a grey area in the collective minds of the general public, because there is so much misinformation surrounding this chemical compound. [3] Its association with the cannabis plant has, historically, discouraged consumers from asking questions about it and deterred medical researchers from studying its properties.

Thankfully, things are starting to change. So, what is CBD? What benefits does it provide when used in its most common form as a medicinal oil? The answers to these questions are crucial, because they can help dispel some of the myths about this wonder substance.

What Is CBD Oil and Where Does It Come From?

CBD is a chemical compound that is extracted from certain varieties of the cannabis plant. It is one of 85 such compounds, but it happens to be the second most abundant.

The most abundant chemical is THC and this is where the distinction between the two becomes really important. [4] THC is the part of the cannabis plant that affects the brain and brings on the high associated with recreational use of the drug. It continues to be illegal in many countries. [5] On the other hand, CBD is something different.

THC and CBD are both what are known as cannabinoids. However, they are separate, distinct properties and CBD has no psychotropic effects on the brain. [6] It cannot get a person high, which is why it is legal in almost every country in the world.

Ingesting CBD as an oil or in any other form is not like smoking marijuana. As a result, it has been used to treat a broad variety of physical and mental ailments.

While scientific research on the impact of CBD oil is still in its infancy, there is compelling evidence to suggest that its use may serve as a powerful treatment for everything from epilepsy to chronic anxiety, diabetes, heart disease, and even cancer. [7]

It is the cultural use of the terms 'marijuana,' 'cannabis,' 'THC,' and 'CBD' that has long caused confusion for consumers. It is common for people to use the words interchangeably, despite the fact that they have very specific meanings. [8] When it comes to the chemical compounds themselves, things are more transparentt. CBD is completely isolated from THC. It is extracted in oil form and often combined with hemp oil extracts to create different concentrations and varieties.

The scientific name for CBD is ‘cannabidiol,’.

Why Is Cannabidiol a Useful Compound?

This is where things get really interesting, because medical researchers have studied cannabinol in many different contexts.

Over the last ten years, its medicinal use has been linked to the treatment and control of many illnesses and physical maladies.

These maladies include multiple sclerosis, bipolar disorder, schizophrenia, convulsions, inflammation, chronic nausea, and more. [9] In fact, one of the most common uses of cannabinol is to treat anxiety, because the substance can bring about a very relaxed feeling, without any of the tension and paranoia linked to smoking cannabis recreationally. [10]

Some researchers have even suggested that cannabidiol has the power to slow down the progression of very aggressive viral strains, like the often fatal MRSA bug.

It is regularly linked to the alleviation of cancer symptoms; though more scientific testing is required. [11] This is true for most of the alleged 'miracle' properties of cannabidiol. The research in this field is still rather young and medical experts are only just beginning to take a closer look. Thus far, findings have been remarkably positive.

What Makes Cannabidiol So Powerful?

On a cellular level, cannabidiol provokes changes within the body by switching on what is known as cannabinoid receptors.

These receptors send diverse of signals around the nervous system. They all have different kinds of impacts, depending on where and how they are activated.

They also account for a large portion of the endocannabinoid system. It regulates everything from appetite to mood, memory, pain tolerance, and more. So, changes made here can have far reaching effects. [12]

Fortunately, scientists have yet to find any negative effects of the medical or recreational use of cannabidiol. While it can induce a state of relaxation, it has no psychotropic influence on the brain and soothes without giving a substance high.

In light of all of its proposed medical benefits, this makes cannabidiol a very valuable property for the medical and health industries. It is legal, can be used in a simple oil form, and it doesn't carry any of the ethical or moral issues associated with drug use.

How Much Medical Research Has Been Done On Cannabidiol?

At this time, there is a lot of conjecture and speculation about the medical applications of cannabidiol and this can make it a challenge to pinpoint the genuine, verifiable information.

There are reliable studies verifying the benefits and use of cannabidiol. These studies involve rigorous tests and established scientific methods.

However, they continue to be in the minority right now and researchers need to keep investing their time and money in cannabidiol studies. With their help, its impact on debilitating conditions can be thoroughly investigated and confirmed.

Surprisingly, what stories about its amazing characteristics don't lack are personal approvals and accounts from regular, ordinary people.

Just googling the words 'cannabidiol' and 'health' bring up a treasure trove of case stories, first-hand accounts, blogs, and articles written by people who claim to be using oils and tinctures to alleviate their symptoms. [13] The important thing to remember is that case studies aren't scientifically verified or peer reviewed. As far as the medical world goes, they can't be considered firm evidence.

Yet, this doesn't mean that they haven't been noticed or explored by scientists.

With so many positive experiences and stories of success, it is hard to dismiss cannabidiol as just another 'natural' medicine that hasn't been subjected to thorough testing.

Besides, medicinal developments like this do often start at ground level, with consumers. Usually, they are looking for an alternative to traditional, commercial treatments. [14] This might be because they are too expensive, they have nasty side effects, or their use leads to addiction.

What Illnesses Is Cannabidiol Currently Being Used to Treat?

If the remarkable medical benefits are to be believed, cannabidiol can solve all of these problems.

It is cost effective when bought in the form of an oil, tincture, or other form.

It has no known side effects and it cannot cause addiction. [15] This is why it is already being used, independently, by patients to treat a plethora of ailments, conditions, and afflictions.

Do remember that, while there is a small amount of research on the use of cannabidiol to treat some of these conditions, this cannot be taken as medical endorsement.

Nicotine Addiction

A number of studies have now linked cannabidiol to the complete cessation or reduction of nicotine consumption.[16] One such trial gave participants a respiratory inhaler. Half were given a device filled with cannabidiol. The other half were given an empty inhaler. They were told to use it every time that they got a craving for nicotine.

After just seven days, the participants inhaling cannabidiol showed a 40% drop in their consumption of nicotine cigarettes.

This is an impressive result and it has encouraged scientists to dig deeper and explore the possibility that cannabidiol could help smokers kick the habit in a natural, soothing way.

The wider implications for the medical industry are huge, particularly if a successful system of treatment were to be established.

At the moment, smoking related diseases cost healthcare services millions of dollars every year.

If used correctly, cannabidiol could reduce this expense by helping smokers to make positive, healthy changes before things like lung disease and cancer set in.

Schizophrenia

The links between cannabidiol use and mental health are some of the strongest. [17] There is no shortage of case studies online about the impact of the compound on mental conditions like anxiety and autism.

For this reason, scientists have long been fascinated by the idea that cannabidiol holds the key to practical, affordable, and effective mental health treatments.

The suggestion that it could alleviate the symptoms of schizophrenia is quite an old one.

In fact, it was one of the very first conditions to be associated with cannabidiol as an alternative medicine.

Thus far, medical trials have been successful, but they need further verification to be accepted in the medical world. In this context, the effects of cannabidiol seem to be relatively short lived, so scientists are looking for a way to extend its influence and create sustainable, long lasting treatments.

Until this happens, the compound can't really be considered a good enough substitute for commercial, pharmaceutical options.

However, it is still used by sufferers – often alongside traditional medicines - to reduce anxiety, increase mental focus, and maintain a sense of calm and equilibrium.

Multiple Sclerosis

In many ways, research on the relationship between multiple sclerosis and cannabidiol represents the cutting edge of medical investigation. [18] If scientists can develop a way to use cannabidiol to soothe the extremely debilitating symptoms of MS, it would be a ground breaking discovery.

What they know so far is that, in mice, the compound can reverse the inflammatory responses that cause the immune system to attack itself.

Within a little over a week, mice treated with cannabidiol demonstrated improved motor functions and a significant reduction in their pain symptoms.

While there may be a long way to go yet before it is made available as a medically approved treatment for MS, progress is being made.

If personal case studies are to be believed, cannabidiol is changing lives for the better right now.

Diabetes

Diabetes has become one of the biggest killers of people in the western world, so doctors are keen to develop a cure or an effective treatment as soon as possible. [19] Once again, cannabidiol tests have been carried out on mice.

This is not to say that the results can be immediately assumed the same for humans, but it is the first step to the road to full testing and approval.

Studies conducted on mice dosed the animals with cannabidiol.

This hindered the production of IL-12, which is a cytokine involved in the onset of several autoimmune diseases. It indicates that cannabidiol could, potentially, be used to either halt or slow the progression of diabetes.

Crucially, this effect has only been observed in mice with Type 1 diabetes. Animals with diabetes caused by poor diet do not respond in the same way, but tests are ongoing.

Chronic Sleep Disorders

Finally, cannabidiol use has also been linked to the alleviation of sleep disorders. [20] Chronic sleep problems are often given much less interest and focus than diseases like diabetes, because they are considered to be a milder issue.

The reality is that a lack of sleep can have disastrous effects on the mind and body. Missing out on just one night of sleep is enough to send a healthy heart rate soaring.

Plus, many of the pharmaceutical treatments for chronic sleep disorders come with a risk of addiction.

The medications can create harmful dependencies and need to be taken more frequently, in larger amounts, to continue to have any effect.

For this reason, a cannabidiol based treatment has great potential. When used as an oil, the compound soothes, relaxes, dispels physical tension, and depending on the strain, also can cause drowsiness.

What Are Some of the Different Ways to Use Cannabidiol?

Cannabidiol is used in a number of different ways to treat many different conditions and ailments. In some cases, it is also used recreationally, but only as a substance that relaxes the mind and sometimes brings about tiredness. [21]

It cannot produce a high or any kind of psychotropic effects. This is why it is not uncommon for cannabidiol to be independently (without official medical consent) prescribed to minors.

While this might sound like a drastic step, it is important to remember all that has been learned about the compound thus far.

It may come from the same plant as THC, but it is not THC. It has no known side effects, other than drowsiness after taking heavier strains.

It has the potential to treat many different types of mental and physical illnesses and this applies to children as well. When it comes to conditions like autism and chronic anxiety, more and more parents are choosing to eschew the conventional, pharmaceutical route and turning to cannabidiol as an alternative. [22]

Ease of use is an important factor here. Cannabidiol is commercially available in the form of tinctures, dietary capsules, pen and 'wand' applicators, and even lip balms and protein powders. [23] Such a variety is helpful for anybody who wants to take that first step and try cannabidiol.

While some people will feel more comfortable with tinctures that are dropped, slowly, into the mouth, others might prefer an external application.

How Much Cannabidiol Is It Safe to Use?

There is no scientific or medical evidence to suggest that consuming cannabidiol, in any quantity, is dangerous. [24] The worst that has been observed is extreme tiredness and, if a person wants to avoid this, they can simply select a lighter strain.

Preferences for the way in which cannabidiol is used are mostly about how much a person wishes to apply at any one time or in a single 'dose.' This is a personal choice.

In order to have complete control and, if desired, a very slow and measured way to use cannabidiol, drops are usually the best choice.

Each drop contains exactly the same amount of the compound, so it is near impossible to unintentionally take more than desired. [25] A more direct way to use it is in the form of liposome sprays. These are more common to experienced users, as they are fast acting and provide a heavier application.

Most liposome products are sprayed directly onto the tongue or the back of the throat.

Even though it is true that no known side effects of cannabidiol exist, it is still important to follow the instructions on these products very carefully. Some varieties, like dietary capsules, require very specific storage conditions or their quality could be compromised.

It must also be noted that in the absence of an official medical endorsement, any consumer using cannabidiol products is doing so at their own risk. It is a really good idea to carry out a small amount of personal research and its uses and applications before making a purchase.

Cannabidiol Capsules

Dietary capsules are one of the easiest ways to consume cannabidiol, as they are just placed on the tongue and swallowed whole like a tablet.

The recommended serving is one capsule per day and this provides approximately 15mg of the compound. Many products actually contain a broader variety of nutrients, alongside cannabidiol, to make them a valuable dietary supplement.

These are all naturally occurring and have no association with synthetic substances.

Capsules tend to be a less intimidating introduction to the world of cannabidiol, because most people have taken supplements like this at some point in their lives; such as flaxseed, cod liver oil, or a multi-vitamin.

They come packaged in a similar manner. Cannabidiol capsules are encased in a soft, pliable glycerine shell. This breaks down in the stomach and releases the substance inside, without causing any irritation whatsoever.

While they are not the best choice for those who struggle to take tablets and pills, they are popular, because they mask the slightly bitter taste of the oil.

They are also highly discreet, which is important for those who feel like the cultural connection between THC and cannabidiol might attract negativity to their use of the product.

Cannabidiol capsules look similar to most other dietary capsules.

They can be carried around in a bag, briefcase, or hold-all and taken in public without attracting any attention.

Plus, each capsule contains the exact same amount of cannabidiol, which makes it easy to control the dosage.

Cannabidiol Tinctures

For even more control over the dose, there are cannabidiol tinctures.

These are most commonly provided as drops, in a small bottle with an internal applicator. In some cases, they are bought as sprays.

Tinctures come in a variety of different strengths, so consumers can start off with a lighter strain and work their way up to bigger does of cannabidiol if they desire. [26] The applicator is quick and easy to use; it is simply extracted from the bottle and the rubber bulb on the top is gently squeezed.

This releases a small amount of cannabidiol and it should be directly applied to the tongue.

This is a popular way to use the substance, particularly for those with experience, as it is quite fast acting. [27] The doses can be kept small and controlled, but the effect is near instant. If a more gradual effect is preferred, capsules are a better option.

One of the most appealing qualities of the cannabidiol tincture is that it lends itself well to substitute flavors. As already mentioned, the taste can be a little bitter and not everybody likes it.

With tinctures, it is easy to mask this taste with other flavors like mint, cinnamon, orange, and even chocolate.

As they are so fast acting, it is common for those with chronic anxiety to turn to cannabidiol tinctures as a form of ‘on the spot’ treatment. [28] It allows them to continue functioning in environments that might otherwise bring on serious attacks. If symptoms start to appear, all that is needed is a few drops of the liquid in the bottle.

Cannabidiol Liposomes

Now, we reach the cutting edge of cannabidiol research and product development.

The term 'liposome' refers to a microscopic bubble that can be filled with a chosen substance. Ordinarily, lifesaving drugs and treatments for conditions like cancer are delivered via these bubbles.

This is because they are made out of the same material as a cell membrane and they leave no synthetic trace in the body whatsoever. [29]

In recent years, liposome sprays have been developed for the use and application of cannabidiol.

They are highly effective and deliver doses faster, more efficiently, and into a deeper part of the cells.

Consequently, for those taking cannabidiol for health reasons, there is no better option. They are very easy to use too.

The tiny bubbles are too small to see with the human eye, so the practical application is as a regular, conventional spray.

It is directed either on the bottom surface on the tongue or at the back of the mouth.

The average liposome spray provides around 5mg of bioavailable cannabidiol per serving.

A recommended dosage is five of these servings, twice every day, though personal preference and use is, of course, encouraged.

The spray bottles are very small and discreet, so they can be carried around in a pocket or small bag.

Cannabidiol Applicator Pen

The cannabidiol oral applicator pen is another relatively new way to ingest the compound. [30] It is increasing in popularity very fast, however, it is largely down to the meteoric rise of things like electronic cigarettes and vape pens.

It actually looks a lot like a vape pen and this makes it another very discreet option for anybody wants to use cannabidiol in public quietly.

Most applicator pens deliver a dose of around 15mg, so they are around the same strength as dietary capsules.

Like tinctures, they are faster acting than capsules, because the cannabidiol is given direct access to the blood stream, via the mouth, as opposed to dissolving in the stomach first.

Applicator pens are easy to use; most have a soft rubber or plastic nib that dispenses the oil into the mouth.

The unique lock and click device allows for careful control, because every individual click delivers the same amount of cannabidiol.

Applicator pens have a number of key benefits, with the most important being their hermetically sealed cartridge.

Cannabidiol oil is very sensitive to light and atmospheric conditions and, if stored incorrectly, it will spoil.

Keeping it in a hygienic, sealed pen extends its freshness and means that it retains its high quality for longer.

Sharing applicator pens is fine, but the recommendation is to invest in a device with a removable, washable nib for hygiene purposes.

Cannabidiol Protein Powders

While the most common way to use cannabidiol is definitely in a liquid form, it is not the only way. There are many reasons why a person might want to avoid oils and sprays.

They might have an aversion to oral capsules and dislike the taste of sprays. They might just be interested in making cannabidiol a more integrated part of their dietary routine.

If this is the case, specially developed protein powders could be the answer. The best formulations have only one or two ingredients. They are all natural and extremely nutritious.

The big advantage of opting for protein powders is that they diversify the use of cannabidiol. They can be put in smoothies, cakes, cereals, muesli, and salads.

They can even be cooked, albeit at low temperatures.

For vegetarians, they represent a safe and healthy way to access the nutritional and medicinal properties of this wonder compound.

If that weren't enough, they also provide protein, iron, magnesium, and omega three fatty acids in abundance. [31]

In fact, the only downside is that some people won't like the taste of cannabidiol in powder form.

One alternative is to switch to capsules or the flavor can be disguised by combining it with other ingredients.

Aside from cooking at high temperatures, there is not much that can be done to spoil cannabidiol protein powders, so experimentation and creativity is very much encouraged for anybody looking to go down this route.

Cannabidiol (Hemp) Seeds

A regular, nutritious dose of cannabidiol may also be provided via the consumption of raw, shelled hemp seeds. Hemp is just the scientific name for the type of cannabis plant that the cannabidiol comes from.

If its seeds are eaten – and this is completely safe – the compound can reach the areas of the body that need nourishing and get to work.

Like protein powders, hemp seeds are an alternative to using cannabidiol oil. For some people, they just feel tidier, healthier, and like a more balanced way to make the substance a part of the daily routine.

Once again, this is all personal preference and, ultimately, the end result is the same.

The advantage of hemp seeds is that they can be consumed with all kinds of regular ingredients. [32] They are particularly appealing on cereals and may be added to smoothies, desserts, salads, and recipes that are cooked at a low temperature.

Bread is a common choice; many hemp seed fans like to sprinkle them in their dough for a warm, nutty taste and a health boost. [33]

Cannabidiol in this form doesn't taste anywhere near as intense as it can do as an oil, so it is a good option for those who struggle with the flavor.

Hemp seeds need to be stored correctly, as they are sensitive to light. It should be noted that they are abundant in a remarkable substance called globulin edistin. It is a basic protein that helps the body fight off sickness and infection. Humans cannot produce this protein naturally within their bodies, so any alternative source is highly valuable and should be prized. [34]

Lip Balms and Salves

Finally, another innovative way to use cannabidiol for health is externally, on the skin or lips. [35] There are all kinds of great creams and lotions on the market, but for a quick and affordable fix, pocket lip balms are great.

The ingredients are natural and contain nothing synthetic, so that the lips are nourished and protected.

According to a number of studies, cannabidiol restores moisture, provides protection from external elements, and increases softness.

Has Medicinal Cannabidiol Ever Actually Worked for Anybody?

It is always important to be open and transparent about scientific research and medical developments.

If cannabidiol is ever going to earn approval as a legitimate medical treatment, it needs to be subjected to rigorous investigation.

It is, therefore, a good idea to look at its positives and negatives with an open mind.

There continues to be a lack of high profile research, for a number of reasons, but the reality is that this situation is changing. It is changing slowly, but progress is being made. [36] In the meantime, the existing scientific research on medicinal cannabidiol and the many personal testimonies of users are the best place to start learning.

There are thousands of first-hand accounts online from people who claim to have cured serious sicknesses by ingesting natural, powerful cannabidiol.

Their stories are compelling, stirring, and highly emotional, because these are people who are claiming to have eliminated some of the most aggressive conditions that we know using nothing but natural plant extracts.

They continue to be added to, with more stories appearing online every week.

They might not have the weight of a peer reviewed journal behind them, but they are worthy of attention.

The doctors and scientists currently testing cannabidiol are the ones on the forefront of this medical movement, but they are not the heart of it.

Real Life Stories

54-Year Old Wife and Mother Beats Lung Cancer with help from CBD Oil

When she was first plagued with sharp, jagged pains around the left hand side of her ribcage, she did what most people would do. [37] She winced, shrugged it off, and hoped it would work itself out. She had recently been in for an intense physical massage and she thought that the movements might have been a bit too firm.

However, the pain continued for a number of days and she started to grow concerned that it might be linked to something more serious.

Unfortunately, she was right and, within days of the pain starting, she had been given a diagnosis of lung cancer.

This is an unimaginable horror, particularly for a mother, but it is one that occurs in thousands of clinics, every single day of the week.

For her, the prognosis was very serious from the outset. Doctors told her that, though the cancer had started in her lung, it had now spread to her lymph nodes and her stomach.

She would only live for a maximum of nine months. In fact, her cancer was so advanced that her specialists didn't consider radiation or chemotherapy to be a viable option.

She was told to return home and enjoy the time that she had left.

However, her daughter was determined to keep searching for a solution.

She scoured the internet for answers and discovered thousands of stories about cancer patients who had treated themselves with cannabidiol oil.

She took the news to her mother and, with nothing left to lose, her mother began dosing herself with small amounts of CBD oil, three times per day. Soon, she had upped the dosage to around two grams each day.

She also embarked on a strict alkalizing clean eating diet, after online advice from former cancer sufferers. [38] Within two to three months, her clinical scans showed something remarkable.

The 5cm tumor inside her left lung had shrunk to 2.1cm. Her cancer ridden lymph nodes had decreased in size and there was no sign of the fluid in the left side of her chest.

At seven months, further scans picked up no indication of cancer in her body.

If asked, she can't really explain what happened to her during this remarkable period of her life. She's no doctor and, even if she was, she'd still find it hard to understand how a simple plant based extract had such a powerful impact on her dying cells.

What she does know is that she's now cancer free and living life to the fullest with her husband and daughter.

The question is, would this still be the case if her daughter had not discovered the wonders of cannabidiol oil?

Two Young Brothers Tackle Autism Symptoms with CBD Oil

A young mother living in California and has two young sons. One is ten years old and has barely spoken for much of his life.

His brother is a little younger at eight years old and has always been more verbal, but he has also had his own difficulties with speaking. Both boys have been diagnosed as severely autistic. They do not have seizures, like many autism sufferers, but life is tough for them at times. [39]

It was until their mother tried cannabidiol oil, their life changed. For a long time, she had been reading stories online and hearing parents talk, mostly in whispers, about the magic of cannabinoids. [40] She was intrigued, if a little surprised, but decided to try CBD for herself, because the situation with her boys had become a concern.

The oldest was almost entirely non-verbal and found it hard to sleep, play with others, go to the toilet, and express his emotions in a healthy way.

His brother functioned a little better, but was dropping behind developmentally and struggling to keep up with his peers. So, she found a specialist willing to prescribe CBD oil (medicinal marijuana use is legal in California) [41] and waited to see if it would help her boys to find a greater joy in life. They have now been given daily doses of CBD oil for three months and a lot of changes have taken place.

Her oldest son has since started talking. He sings songs, counts, and gestures loudly at objects. He can speak about what he wants to eat, what he likes to draw, and what type of music makes him want to dance around.

Gone are the screaming fits and the attempts to take his clothes off in inappropriate situations. He still has upsets, from time to time, but his mood has been transformed.

His younger brother is not far behind; he's talking more, going to the toilet by himself, and learning how to express his emotions in a calm, sensible manner.

The mother has had mixed reactions from families in her community. There are other parents of autistic children who understand her actions or even use CBD oil to treat their own children.

There are others who find it harder to get past its association with THC and cannot understand why she should dose her children with it. In response to this, she assures people that she has done her research and she has a doctor review the boys and their progress every three months.

CBD oil has transformed her sons and she wouldn't have it any other way. Now, she is taking her learning further and is interested in finding out more about the medicinal benefits of cannabidiol. She refers people to a recent study which found that the use of cannabinoids actually leads to the growth of new nerve cells in the hippocampus. There is evidence to suggest that this might aid the preservation of memories in later years. [42]

Parents of Severely Epileptic Boy Treat Seizures with CBD Oil

[43] In May 2016, the wonders of CBD oil were given a rare moment in the spotlight by the mainstream media. CNN published a very interesting story about a family in Haifa, Israel. [44] The birth of their son was in 2014. It was meant to be a moment of unbelievable joy, but things didn't go as expected.

The child was born unconscious. Just a few hours later, he would have the first of many severe epileptic seizures.

At only hours old the newborn was rushed to an emergency unit and spent the first week of his life heavily sedated to prevent the seizures from killing him.

He was eventually allowed home and for the next six months, his parents prayed that the episodes would stop.

At its worst, his epilepsy caused him to have dozens of seizures every day. He was still just a tiny little baby as well; taken in and out of hospital for countless exams, tests, and treatments.

The baby would later be diagnosed with cerebral palsy, on top of his epilepsy.

He is severely brain damaged. In 2015, after many months of unsuccessful treatments with nasty side effects, the father heard about medical marijuana and, in particular, CBD oil. He submitted a request for a dispensary license to the Israeli Ministry of Health. In Israel, it is legal to use cannabis medicinally if you have a license. It is sold, from approved growers, at a fixed rate price and amounts are strictly controlled. [45]

The government is keen to remind citizens that there are still vast gaps in our knowledge of marijuana and that they take it at their own risk.

However, it also agrees that many debilitating medical conditions can be soothed and alleviated with its careful use. [46] The license that the father has allows him to give his son a micro dose (just a few drops) of CBD oil every day. He has been doing this for a year and the seizures have stopped.

According to the father, this happened around three weeks after he started to treat his son with CBD oil. Though life is still hard – his son will always be severely disabled – he no longer has daily fits and can interact with his parents.

His quality of life has been significantly improved thanks to the use of cannabidiol. Yet, there are plenty of people who are still very opposed to such treatments, particularly for the very young.

Were these parents right to self-treat their infant child with a cannabinoid? Is it ever safe to give a baby a derivative of the cannabis plant?

It is a tough question, but one which medical researchers in Israel have been pondering for some time. As Dr. Kramer, from the Child Epilepsy Unit in Tel Aviv is keen to point out, 'If a severely epileptic child is not a suitable candidate for surgery, there aren't really any other conventional medical solutions.' [47]

UFC Heavyweight Defends Use of Healing CBD Vape Pen

A UFC fighter is currently embroiled in a very public debate about the medicinal use of cannabidiol. [48]

The 31-year old fighter was defeated by an Irish champion this August, in one of most anticipated bouts of the year.

Both before and after the fight, he was pictured puffing on a vape pen. When asked what was inside, he didn't hesitate to explain that it was medicinal CBD oil and he uses it to help him heal.

At the time, the comment didn't attract much attention, but the UFC has now ordered that he put down the pen or stay outside of the cage. [49] Considering the fact that cannabidiol does not have the psychotropic qualities of THC and cannot get a person high, nor improve their physical performance, is this fair to demand?

Moreover, is this fighter right to think that this natural plant extract can actually help wounds to heal faster?

It is an interesting thought and the fighter has broken new ground just by being a high profile public figure happy to admit that he uses it.

He is keen to point out that he passes all of the mandatory drug tests before bouts and that his use of cannabidiol is not for performance, but for restoration. Surprisingly, he is supported by the might of the US Department of Health and Human Services. In 1999, it patented cannabinoids as antioxidants and neuro-protectants. [50]

In other words, it appears to be the perfect medicinal response to a job which lists brain injury as one of its biggest risks. Cannabidiol has the ability to limit neurological damage caused by trauma or strokes. [51] It can minimize the immediate impact of temporary blockages of blood to the brain, without compromising it in the way that THC might.

As an experienced UFC fighter, he is well aware of this, so is it fair for the compound to be banned outright?

For the time being, he has agreed to put down his CBD vape pen in order to stay in the cage. It remains to be seen, however, whether he will contest the decision at a later date.

At the very least, his personal and public use of the substance will hopefully get people talking about why it is still so controversial.

We have known for many years that THC and cannabidiol are completely separate entities, so it is time to bring the debate about CBD to the forefront of public consciousness.

A Survivor Becomes A Leading Expert in the Use of CBD

Her name is well known to long term users of cannabidiol in the United States. [52] She is a leading authority within the CBD oil industry and owns a company which manufactures some of the highest quality extracts anywhere in the world. [53] It is fair to say that she knows her stuff. There's a good reason for this too. It wasn't so long ago that she was fighting a medical battle that conventional pharmaceuticals just couldn't touch.

Her experiences with serious illnesses and the journey back to health inspired her to take what she had learned and use it not just to help others, but to save their lives.

Today, her company is considered to be the gold standard for whole plant cannabis extracts and the entrepreneur is on a mission to open eyes and minds. [54] It all started, however, with an autoimmune disease and a pharmaceutical prescription that changed everything.

For many years, she was gravely sick with an autoimmune disorder. She was almost completely housebound and, in her own words, had a very poor quality of life.

As her disease was a rare one, doctors weren't sure how best to treat it and gave her a plethora of pills and medications.

If they were effective, the results didn't last for long and she continued to struggle with extreme pain and inflammation.

Yet, it wasn't until a risky encounter with a new prescription that she decided there had to be another way.

In short, she almost died from complications caused by the pharmaceuticals prescribed to her. It was at this point that she began to research the benefits of medical cannabis, particularly in regards to pain relief.

As she was confined to her house, she occupied most of her free time reading studies on cannabinoids and investigating claims of cured cancer and vanishing tumors. She found them convincing enough to start experimenting with unfertilized cannabis plant extracts.

While she cannot cure her affliction with cannabidiol, after years of dosing, she manages to live mostly pain free and is no longer housebound. She has regained her quality of life and now runs a modern, biodynamic farming operation. [55] She is committed to growing and producing cannabidiol and other cannabinoids in the most natural, organic way possible.

Her company uses nothing but fully trimmed, female unfertilized cannabis sativa plants with known and controlled genetics.

To put it simply, she knows where every plant comes from and how it has been grown. It is a firm commitment to the values that she took up when first experimenting with CBD oil.

Being so sick, she knew that making the wrong move could spell disaster, so she was extremely discerning about what she put in her body. She then carried this idea with her as she set up the company; if it isn't good enough for her, it isn't good enough for her customers either. Yet, there is also another important reason why quality is such a big priority.

She believes that, in order for cannabidiol and other cannabinoids to ever be looked upon seriously by the pharmaceutical and medical industries, quality, consistency, and potency must be managed meticulously.

When researchers and scientists finally do lift their heads and ask to know more, she stresses the importance of being able to offer them clear, verifiable data.

She has plenty of it too, in the form of glowing testimonials from clients with cancer, autoimmune disorders, Lyme disease, Huntington's, Parkinson's and more.

Grandfather of Nine Beats Cancer 'Breaking Bad' Style

In 2014, popular UK newspaper the Daily Mail published a story that got people talking. [56] It told the tale of a man who was confronted by a terminal cancer diagnosis in 2009. [57] The first sign of trouble came after he collapsed at work and doctors immediately sent him for a series of tests. They found an advanced stage of cancer in his liver and told him that, without surgical intervention, he wouldn't live more than 3-4 months.

As a grandfather, the thought of not taking any action was terrifying, so he agreed to go ahead with an emergency liver transplant to try and remove the cancerous cells.

All seemed well until the year 2012, when he was told that his cancer had returned. Not only that, but it has become so aggressive that doctors weren't willing to offer him chemotherapy or radiation. They prescribed morphine and advised him to go home and spend time with his wife and grandchildren.

They underestimated his will to survive. He wasted no time diving into the world of alternative treatments and herbal therapies. After much research, he chanced upon the well-known documentary 'Run from the Cure.' It is a much celebrated account of a Canadian and his own battle with cancer. [58] His claims that he cured his disease with the use of cannabidiol and his story is highly regarded by those who regularly use cannabinoids for pain relief and the management of chronic sickness.

The grandfather was keen to give CBD oil a try for himself, because there was simply nothing to lose. He began dosing himself in April 2013. It took just three days for the excruciating pain in his body to vanish. In his own words, he was 'utterly amazed.' After 2-3 months of taking CBD oil – a point at which doctors had expected the man to already be dead – he began coughing up blood.

Unsurprisingly, this caused him some concern, but he now believes that the blood contained dead cancer cells and his body was simply ejecting them.

It sounds remarkable, but a recent biopsy has confirmed that he no longer has cancer. A spokesperson from the hospital where he was a patient at has also verified this and stated that he has received no conventional cancer treatments since his original transplant in 2009. He is cancer free, fit, and healthy and it has nothing to do with traditional medical interventions.

Can it really be just a coincidence that his sickness disappeared after he started regularly taking CBD oil?

Well, medical experts are being very cagey on the subject, which is to be expected. This man is from the UK, where even the medicinal use of cannabis or cannabis plant extracts is not legal.

This means that he had to break the law to both acquire CBD oil and, later, to grow his own plants. It earned him the nickname, in the papers, of Walter White; hence the Breaking Bad association. [59] Naturally, doctors are trying to discourage others from following his example, but is this the right thing to do? It certainly makes sense to ask whether such an attitude is actually putting lives at risks.

Crucially, a study published by the University of East Anglia has found evidence that cannabinoids can halt the growth of cancerous cells.

According to researchers, the results could lead to the creation of more effective cancer treatments in the future, but they are in the minority right now. In order to start treating patients with CBD oil and other cannabinoids, more studies need to be carried out. [60]

Cancer Sufferer from Australia Finds Miracle Cure in Cannabis

This is the story of yet another cancer sufferer who found the answer in cannabinoids, rather than conventional medical treatments. [61] It involves an Australian lady, in her mid-fifties. She recently made headlines in her country after going public with details about her lung cancer battle. She was originally diagnosed with stage four lung cancer, which is the most aggressive and pervasive. It is very rare for cancer this advanced to be treated with radiotherapy or chemotherapy.

Like most other patients who get to this stage, the woman was told that she only had months to live and more treatments would only rob her of this time. For a while, she prayed.

She had never so much as touched a cigarette in her life, the fact that she had lung cancer seemed awfully unfair. She felt despondent and was ready to give in, until her daughter persuaded her to do some research on medicinal marijuana.

Now, it must be pointed out that the lady in this story used both CBD oil and plant extracts containing THC, which are still illegal in many countries.

While both are linked to remarkable health benefits, cannabidiol (or CBD oil) is the most likely to become an approved medical treatment in the future. It cannot get a person high, because it doesn't have any psychotropic effects and, therefore, it isn't really a recreational drug. On the other hand, THC is the compound that recreational users depend upon to produce their 'high.'

The use of THC is illegal in Australia and even the medicinal use of cannabis is prohibited. In fact, so taboo is the subject that the woman in the story has withheld her name. She was forced to break the law to acquire her CBD and THC compounds and is, naturally, keen to keep her full identity out of the papers. [62] This doesn't detract from the incredible things that happened to her after she started dosing herself with cannabis plant extracts.

Within three months, all traces of her lung cancer had disappeared. She has actually produced before and after PET scans to prove this and they make for very interesting viewing indeed. It must also be pointed out that, alongside her doses, she stuck to a strict sugar free diet and received near constant advice from CBD oil support and advocacy groups. [63] Even still, for all of the cancerous cells to vanish within the space of three months is nothing short of miraculous.

In fact, the only real disappointment in this tale is the response of her doctor, who despite acknowledging the absence of cancer cells, told her that the results couldn't last. In short, she told a healthy woman to expect to be dying again soon. Ultimately, there is no way to know if she'll turn out to be right or not, but for now, this Aussie survivor is cancer free and ready to start living the rest of her life.

CBD Oil Leaves 3 Year Old Boy Almost Entirely Seizure Free

[64] In Oklahoma, a number of parents and CBD oil support groups have spent the last few years campaigning for changes to laws on medicinal marijuana. [65] It follows a series of remarkable success stories involving young children with severe epilepsy. One of these youngsters is a three-year-old. After being dosed with CBD oil, he went from suffering a heart-breaking ten seizures every single day to only five. This change occurred over the course of just a couple of months and his mother is convinced that cannabidiol is the reason.

By working closely with a neurologist, she has been able to safely treat her son with CBD oil and the family has now reached a point where he is almost entirely seizure free.

He has learned to sit up for the first time ever and he is even beginning to crawl unaided. The convulsions that used to consume his short life are a blessed rarity, compared to their past frequency, and he can go several days without one.

According to his mother, his progress is unbelievable. Where he was once silent, he can now call for his parents. Where he used to be unresponsive, he is now more alert and can engage with those around him.

The use of CBD oil has supported his mental and physical development and, even though he will never be as fully able as other children, there is a chance for him to live a happy, contented life.

This is something that comes up again and again in these success stories; a simple, pure appreciation for the power of natural medicines.

It is a sentiment that CBD oil critics like to dismiss as unreliable. They want only the medical facts. They will only entertain scientifically verified research. It is a practical, logical stance, because the fight to raise awareness of cannabidiol and its health benefits can only be grounded in absolutes and certainties. However, if medical science does recognize the value of CBD oil one day, it will be these very human stories that they use to prove their case to the general public. [66]

Utah Family Calls for CBD Oil Treatment to Be Approved

There is a family living in Orem, Utah, who have had what most of us would describe as a terrible kind of luck. [67] They have three daughters. They are all afflicted with an extremely painful disorder called Metachromatic Leukodystrophy (or MLD). Sadly, their eldest daughter was killed by the neurodegenerative disease and her heartbroken parents have been left terrified for the future of their two remaining girls.

MLD is an inherited condition that affects only one in 40,000 people in the western world. It is a particularly nasty sickness with no known cure and there is surely nothing worse on this earth than having to watch a child suffer with it; not just any child, but your own.

They know this better than anybody, because both surviving daughters are now showing signs of the illness. It involves the gradual deterioration of cognitive and motor function. In short, both the brain and the ability to move are stolen.

MLD patients must withstand very painful symptoms, particularly as their disease nears its end and there are few conventional treatments that can ease this. [68] It is difficult to imagine how an adult would feel receiving such a diagnosis, but they were given the news when their daughter was just thirteen years old. She died only two years later and her parents, being aware that this could happen to their other children, are determined to walk a different path this time.

In Utah, the medicinal use of cannabidiol is prohibited, but they have decided that the risk is worth the reward if it can help their daughters manage the painful symptoms of MLD.

When the second oldest daughter began to have seizures, suffer from depression, and experience memory loss, they put her on an experimental regimen of CBD oil. At first, they were both highly skeptical and scared that they might cause more harm. However, within a week, the violent seizures had vanished.

She continues to be very sick. As already mentioned, there is no known cure for MLD and the future doesn't look hopeful.

Yet, it is no small feat that CBD oil is helping them to reduce the pain that their child is experiencing. If she is certain to die, they want her to live out her last years with as much happiness and joy as possible and cannabidiol is making that a possibility.

The sad news is that, in being so vocal about their adoption of alternative therapies, they have attracted a lot of negative attention from the press and the law.

Now, they are merely hoping that a little compassion will encourage the authorities to turn a blind eye and allow them to act in their capacity as parents and caregivers.

Terminally Ill Dad Says 'No' to Tumor with CBD Oil

A terminally ill father with a brain tumor claims to have stopped its growth altogether by dosing himself with cannabidiol. [69] A man from Ireland was given a shocking diagnosis after doctors discovered cancerous cells in his brain tissue. He was told that he'd be lucky to live another year and that around nine months was more likely.

Now, it's two year later and he is not just alive, he's currently dazzling medical experts with what appears to be at a complete halt in the progression of his tumor. This is highly unusual, as brain cancer is extremely aggressive and patients are rarely expected to live longer than a few years at best.

Yet, his doctors have confirmed that the tumor, while still present, has stopped growing.

They cannot tell him if the cancer will get worse in the future, but conventional treatments have been paused because there's no longer any need for them.

They are now investigating the reasons why the tumor is dormant and he is convinced that he has the answer. He has been taking CBD oil for around two years and he believes that it is responsible for preventing the cancerous cells from spreading.

The problem is that the laws surrounding the medicinal and therapeutic use of cannabinoids are still very murky in Ireland. For the most part, use of the compounds even for heath purposes is strictly controlled. However, there are a number of pharmaceutical products that do contain them;

they include treatments for multiple sclerosis. [70] For this man, any legal risk involved with acquiring and consuming cannabidiol is acceptable, because there is no way to know if the tumor would start growing again without it.

In the past, he has undergone both brain surgery and bouts of radiation therapy, but nothing affected the tumor until he began dosing with CBD oil.

This has encouraged him to become a vocal advocate for the full legalization of medicinal marijuana. In his own words, 'there's nothing scary about people who are using it [cannabis plant extracts] to live. They are not on the street selling drugs. They aren't hurting anybody.'

He is a member of the End Our Pain campaign, which is calling for the UK government to decriminalize medical cannabis. [71] They allege that more than a million people in Great Britain would physically and mentally benefit from such a development.

Regardless of its impact, he vows to keep using cannabidiol for the rest of his life. He hopes that, in time, the compound will cause the tumor to start shrinking. If this happens and it becomes small enough, he'll be a candidate for chemotherapy and may one day see a cancer free future.

The Remarkable Story of 'Charlotte's Web'

Currently, the highest profile and easily accessible CBD oil in America is called Charlotte's Web. [72] It is a cannabis plant extract that contains trace amounts of THC (a legal quantity) and a high proportion of cannabidiol. [73] It is sold, lawfully, as a dietary supplement throughout the US and it has just been made legal in the United Kingdom too. [74] For anybody who has ever taken CBD oil for medicinal purposes, this product is the Holy Grail.

It was one of the first and it broke new ground. Yet, while many people are aware of Charlotte's Web and the various benefits that it can provide, fewer people know how it came to be in the first place.

In 2006, a family grew and their two-year-old son became a big brother to twins, one was named Charlotte.

The family was naturally delighted and both babies seemed healthy, happy, and perfectly normal.

That is until around three months after the birth when baby Charlotte had her first seizure.

It lasted a staggering thirty minutes and she was urgently admitted to hospital.

Doctors were reluctant to give a diagnosis and, after checking her out, sent the family home with the reassurance that it was probably an anomaly.

They were wrong. Charlotte suffered a longer, more severe seizure just a week later.

Over the next four months, she had multiple seizures per week, with some lasting as long as four hours.

Life for them became a near constant rotation of hospital visits and a growing sense of fear for the future of their child. It was made worse by the fact that doctors still couldn't spot the source of the problem in scans or blood tests. They continued to tell them that the convulsions were a phase.

Eventually, as her condition worsened, medical experts were forced to consider the possibility of Dravet Syndrome. This is a rare and severe form of epilepsy which cannot be controlled with medication. [75] The only pharmaceutical option is to dull the brain with barbiturates. This had the effect of disrupting Charlotte's mental and physical development, even while it reduced the severity of her episodes. By the age of two, it was clear that a more drastic intervention would be needed if they didn't want to lose their daughter forever.

The father carried out his own research and got in contact with the family of a Dravet sufferer in California. This young boy was being successfully treated with cannabidiol.

At this point, Charlotte had lost the ability to walk, talk, and eat, so the situation was very urgent indeed.

She was experiencing three hundred seizures every week. Despite being a lifelong critic of marijuana use, she agreed to give it a try after doctors admitted that they had exhausted all of their treatment ideas.

The results were near instant. After dosing Charlotte with a small amount of CBD oil, she went an hour without her customary three, four, or five seizures. She didn't have another episodes for the next seven days.

At six years old, the youngster was showing a truly unbelievable amount of positive progress. Her fits had fallen to 2-3 per month and they mostly occurred while sleeping. This was the result after just four milligrams of CBD oil for every pound of her body weight. [76]

She sings, dances, plays with her friends, and enjoys life in all of the ways that a healthy little girl is supposed to do. Her parents are aware that she'll need to be constantly monitored and constantly medicated – in one way or another – for the rest of her days, but it is a small price to pay for the ability to walk, talk, and speak like everybody else. In a heart-warming twist to the tale, the CBD formula that they originally used to bring their daughter back from the brink was later named 'Charlotte's Web.' [77]

Should I Start Taking Cannabidiol to Treat My Illness?

After such an intensive exploration of real life triumphs and successes, it is pertinent to ask whether or not people currently suffering from terminal or chronic diseases should now consider dosing themselves with cannabidiol.

Unfortunately, the answer is a very complicated one and it isn't the same for everybody. For a start, the legal status of the compound seems to be constantly in flux, even as it becomes more widely available.

Certainly, outside the United States, the laws surrounding its use can be difficult to understand at times.

Then, of course, there is the fact that only a small portion of medical experts are happy to publically endorse the medicinal use of cannabidiol.

From all that has been learned so far, it should be clear that this doesn't necessarily mean that they don't believe in its power. Nevertheless, few doctors and neurologists are willing to publically support its adoption as a medical treatment, despite compelling evidence.

It must be remembered then that choosing to medicate or treat with cannabidiol is a risk. Ingesting and consuming it won't produce any nasty side effects, but there are no medical guarantees that it will relieve pain, soothe symptoms, or perform better than conventional drugs.

There are only these testimonies and the thousands of others like them. It is entirely up to the individual to decide if and how to incorporate them into their own lives.

Before experimenting with cannabidiol, it is a good idea to do a small amount of personal research on the various different forms available and where to source reliable products.

Only buy from licensed vendors that can provide information about where the cannabidiol has come from and how it was grown.

Start with small amounts, in order to learn how to control the dosage, and if possible, speak with a doctor or other medical professional about the potential physical responses.

What Are Medical Experts Saying About the Use of Cannabidiol?

Currently, there are more medical trials and studies being conducted on the use of cannabidiol than there has ever been before. [78] This is representative of a shift in attitudes. It is becoming less taboo for scientists and researchers to suggest that cannabis plant extracts might have medicinal and therapeutic benefits. The widespread availability of CBD oil products like Charlotte's Web – which is now legally sold in the United Kingdom as well – is a clear indication that things are changing.

The world is becoming receptive to the wonders of cannabidiol. Nevertheless, the process is a slow one, as most scientific revolutions are. It takes a long time to reverse decades of negative press and harmful stereotypes and it won't be done overnight. [79] What is important is that the scientific study of cannabidiol continues to move forward and researchers produce more verifiable, peer reviewed results. Though the real life stories of cancer and epilepsy survivors may be compelling, they must come second to medical facts.

There are thousands of fascinating case studies on the use of cannabidiol that have been published online and in medical journals.

To really get a feel for how broad its impact might be, it is necessary to take a closer look at a number of examples. The following section will, therefore, summarize some of the most recent scientific, social, medical, and therapeutic developments on the benefits of cannabidiol.

Case Studies

Cannabidiol Reduces Psychosis in Patients with Parkinson's disease

In 2009, the British Association of Psychopharmacology published a study on the effects of cannabidiol on levels of psychosis in patients with Parkinson's disease. [80] The treatment of such symptoms has long been a topic of interest for clinicians, as they can severely degrade quality of life for sufferers. Advanced psychosis involves visual and auditory hallucinations and, very often, the patient becomes catatonic. [81]

The study involved the use of an open label pilot design. Six outpatients (four men and two women) diagnosed with Parkinson's and psychosis were given variable doses of cannabidiol.

This was combined with their usual therapies. All patients were initially dosed with 150mg of cannabidiol per day. For some, the amount was gradually increased over the course of the four-week study.

The aim was to determine whether the supposed neuroprotective and antipsychotic properties of cannabidiol could have an impact on psychosis symptoms.

The researchers were not only on the lookout for positive changes.

Any negative side effects or consequences were also recorded, so as to learn more about how safe it is to use cannabidiol for therapeutic purposes.

After four weeks, all patients were evaluated using the approved Brief Psychiatric Rating Scale [82] and the Parkinson Psychosis Questionnaire. [83]

The results show that, according to these credentials, the symptoms of psychosis were significantly reduced in all patients after cannabidiol treatments.

No adverse side effects were observed and the CBD doses did not have any negative impacts or impair motor functions. The researchers, therefore, concluded that cannabidiol may be a safe, effective, and tolerable treatment for the control of psychosis symptoms in Parkinson's patients. [84]

Cannabis Plant Extract Can Help Kick Recreational Marijuana Addiction

This is a fascinating study and one that really strikes at the heart of scientific taboos still surrounding the use of cannabidiol. [85] A study published in the Journal of Clinical Pharmacy and Therapeutics has discovered that this cannabis plant extract can actually help people addicted to recreational marijuana kick the habit. It sounds remarkable, because they're both from the same plant. So, how can one be beneficial and the other destructive?

Well, the debate on exactly how harmful regular THC use really is – or whether it is harmful at all – continues to rage on, but most doctors and experts agree that heavy, prolonged consumption makes cessation difficult.

This is because moving from ingesting a lot of THC to ingesting no THC produces intense withdrawal symptoms. As with many other recreational drugs, this can make it hard to quit. Withdrawal symptoms include anxiety, insomnia, loss of appetite, migraines, irritability, and restlessness. [86]

Tolerance to cannabis and cannabis withdrawal is believed to be a result of the THC desensitizing CB receptors. The study aimed to find out if cannabidiol could have an effect on the severity of symptoms and, potentially, make it easier for heavy THC users to quit. It observed the case of a 19-year old woman suffering from cannabis withdrawal symptoms. She was treated with cannabidiol for ten consecutive days and kept under observation.

At the end of the study, her anxiety and dissociative symptoms had vanished.

Thus, the researchers concluded that cannabidiol can be an effective treatment for cannabis withdrawal symptoms and may have value for those trying to control their addiction to THC. It is important to point out that this study did only involve one individual, so it cannot be considered as reliable as trials featuring much larger sample sizes. It has been replicated on a number of occasions, however, and the results have been similarly positive. [87]

Cannabidiol Slows the Growth of Breast Cancer Cells in Mice

The Journal of Pharmacology published details, in 2006, of an Italian study on the impact of cannabinoids on breast cancer cells. [88] The relationship between cancer and cannabidiol is one of the most contested, but also one of the most consistently affirmed by both real life testimony and medical research. After so much data has been produced on the link between the two, it is all but impossible to deny that such a connection does exist.

While we may not yet fully understand why cannabidiol changes the behavior of cancer cells, we do know that its potential as a future treatment could be huge.

The Italian study observed a sample of mice, with artificially implanted human breast cancer cells beneath their skin. The mice were dosed with one of five natural cannabinoids (including THC and cannabidiol). The cannabidiol was, by some margin, the most powerful of the five.

It slowed the growth of the human cancer cells. It did not kill or eradicate them, but it did significantly impede their development.

Crucially, cannabidiol also greatly reduced the chance of lung metastases as a result of the breast cancer cells. In short, it stopped the disease from spreading and becoming terminal.

This left the researchers in no doubt that cannabidiol requires further testing as a possible treatment for cancer.

The study was followed by another, in 2011, which built upon its findings by discovering that cannabidiol induces a process called autophagy. [89] It does not kill the cancer cells directly, but it works to create conditions within the body that are hostile to them. For instance, it may block access to essential nutrients or other factors needed for growth. In some cases, this then leads to apoptosis; a form of programmed cell destruction. [90]

Cannabidiol May Reduce Seizures in Children and Young Adults

The importance of developing effective treatments for epilepsy becomes even clearer with the realization that close to a third of all patients has a treatment resistance that forms. [91] This means that they couldn't be given conventional medications to alleviate the symptoms. These people are extremely difficult for clinicians to manage and, in the most severe cases; quality of life is significantly impaired.

A very recent (2016) study published by The Lancet Neurology Journal aimed to find out if cannabidiol could be an effective alternative treatment for this kind of epilepsy. [92] It focused particularly on the treatment of children and young adults. To achieve the objective, researchers observed a sample of 214 patients aged between 1-30 years. All had either severe, intractable, childhood onset, or treatment resistant epilepsy.

All participants were already receiving anti-convulsant medications. They were kept under observation at a number of specialist centers across the USA.

Each was given an oral dose of cannabidiol (2-5mg) every day.

This was then gradually increased until intolerance or a maximum of 25mg per day.

The researchers then recorded any changes in the frequency and intensity of their seizures.

The results show a median reduction in monthly motor seizures of 5% (or 36 individual seizures) over a twelve-week period.

However, these positive effects were mainly limited to patients with the most treatment resistant forms of epilepsy. This led researchers to conclude that, while cannabidiol may have potential as a treatment for severe epilepsy, more research is required before this impact can be deemed representative of a wider population. [93]

Colon Cancer Cells Slowed by Cannabinol Treatment

The Journal of Molecular Medicine contains details of a study conducted on the in vivo effect of cannabidiol treatments on colon cancer cells. [94] It observed a sample of mice that had been artificially implanted with human cancer cells. The animals were seen to develop tumors and other symptoms commonly associated with the growth of cancerous tissues.

However, once the mice were dosed with cannabidiol, the numbers of ACF (abnormal cells within the colon), polyps, and tumors were reduced.

This was combined with a significant increase in the production of caspase-3, which plays a vital role in cell apoptosis (cell destruction). It is an important finding, because many cancers – including colon cancer – have shown an ability to evade this process. Across the colorectal carcinoma cell lines, cannabidiol protected human DNA from sustaining oxidative damage.

It helped to regulate the healthy function of the endocannabinoid system and slowed the development of cancerous tissues.

This led the researchers to conclude that cannabidiol could have great potential as a treatment for colon cancer, as it clearly demonstrates chemopreventive properties. Cannabidiol has, for many years, been used by terminally ill patients who no longer have access to effective conventional treatments. [95]

This is usually the case if a tumor is in a dangerous position (in the brain, for example) or if treating the cancer with chemotherapy or radiotherapy would not have much of an impact. In this situations, cannabidiol is one of very few methods that a patient can try.

It is often turned to out of desperation, but the results speak for themselves. Plus, similar medical trials have been carried out on breast, neck, and liver cancer cells; the majority have produced positive outcomes and recommended that cannabidiol be tested and investigated further.

Researchers Discover Cannabidiol Has Anti-Anxiety Effect

The 2004 Neuropsychopharmacology Journal contains an interesting investigation into the impact of cannabidiol on the anxiolytic capacities of the human brain. [96] The aim was to find out whether changes to regional cerebral blood flow – brought about by cannabidiol consumption – could have a positive impact on anxiety levels. The relationship between anxiety and cannabidiol is a fairly old one.

Despite the common assumption being that it must provoke paranoia, as THC sometimes does, there is actually an abundance of evidence to suggest that cannabidiol is very soothing to the brain.

To test this theory, the researchers measured the regional cerebral blood flow of ten healthy male volunteers. They did this with the use of functional neuroimaging tools. The sample group was split into two categories of five and observed two times, each a week apart.

During the first observation, they were given either an oral dose (400mg) of cannabidiol or they were given a placebo. The study used a double blind design.

Ninety minutes after ingestion of the CBD, all participants were sent for brain scans. They were asked questions, during the procedure, according to the Visual Analogue Mood Scale.

On the second occasion, the process was repeated, but the categories were switched around (the researchers were unware of the order of this method). So, over the course of the study, all of the patients received one dose of cannabidiol, but at different times. The brain scans taken after ingestion of CBD showed a significant reduction in anxiety and a substantial boost to mental sedation.

The placebo produced none of these changes. Therefore, it is reasonable to suggest that cannabidiol does have a soothing effect on the brain and could, potentially be used to treat anxiety disorders.

Cannabidiol Proposed as a Potential Treatment for FIRES Syndrome

The medical term FIRES won't mean much to most people. Its slightly wordier moniker – acute encephalitis with refractory repetitive partial seizures – probably means even less. [97] This is because it is a very rare disease that doctors are still trying to get to grips with. It affects a small number of children who are recovering from a serious fever. Instead of getting healthier and stronger, their intellectual capacity declines and they begin to have epileptic episodes. [98]

The most frightening thing about FIRES (or febrile related epilepsy syndrome) is that nobody really knows why it develops.

Scientists think that it could be caused by a number of different things, such as infection or genetics, but they don't know for sure.

This makes the condition very difficult to treat and, while medications can be used to reduce the severity of the seizures, they are not usually all that effective.

This is why, in September 2016, the Journal of Child Neurology published a study on the impact of cannabidiol as a potential treatment for FIRES.

The aim was to determine whether the plant extract has a positive effect on the severity and frequency of seizures for children diagnosed with FIRES.

It involved a total of seven infants, all of whom had failed to respond to conventional treatments, like antiepileptic medications and other therapies.

The children were, instead, dosed with cannabidiol.

It should be noted that all participants were in an acute or chronic phase of illness. In short, they were very sick and their symptoms were either life threatening or very close to being so.

One child died during the course of the study, but this is not thought to be related to the cannabidiol treatments. Six of the seven participants demonstrated significantly less severe and less frequent seizures after dosage.

As the treatments continued, five of the children showed a greatly enhanced ability to walk unaided.

One child was able to walk with assistance. Four of the children started to talk. These are quite dramatic results and the researchers were happy to conclude that cannabidiol could be used as a safe treatment for the symptoms of FIRES, particularly in relation to patients who are not responding well to conventional treatments. [99]

Scientists Studying Mental Health Discover That Cannabidiol Reduces the Memory

Impairment and Paranoia Associated with THC Consumption **[100]**

The relationship between cannabidiol and THC has always been a complex one. For many years, both compounds were demonized as a result of unchecked recreational use.

After THC was made illegal across large swathes of the planet, it became hard for the general public to distinguish between the two and cannabidiol was mistakenly linked with the psychotropic effects of its edgier, riskier sister extract.

This is still happening today, but things are gradually changing. We now know that cannabidiol and THC are completely separate substances and that the former does not produce any kind of recreational high. [101]. It is less clear what kind of impact the two have on one another. This is what scientists were trying to determine when they carried out a study on the mental health effects of both THC and CBD.

The study involved two groups of people.

All were dosed with 1.5mg of pure, intravenous THC.

However, only one of the groups was given an additional 600mg cannabidiol dose before being asked to take the THC. The main reason for this is because researchers have long suspected that pre-dosing with cannabidiol might soothe and reduce the effects of the THC; particularly paranoia and memory problems. [102]

The cannabidiol dose (or placebo) was delivered 210 minutes before the THC dose. The results showed a very small reduction in PANSS scores [103] for the CBD group.

However, this wasn't enough of a difference to be considered significant.

On the other hand, clinically significant psychotic symptoms were noticeably less likely for this group. Levels of paranoia were also smaller and episodic memory was more efficient.

The findings clearly support the proposal that cannabidiol counteracts some of the more harmful mental effects of THC.

Epilepsy Study Shows That Cannabidiol Can Boost the Impact of Anti-Seizure Drug Clobazam

[104] In 2015, the highly regarded Epilepsia journal featured a very interesting study on the drug-drug interaction between cannabidiol and Clobazam, which is a very common anticonvulsant treatment [105]. The aim of the study was to test whether or not the two substances would affect one another because they are metabolized within the same cytochrome pathway [106]. For researchers, this shared link indicated a strong possibility of some kind of engagement.

The study involved a total of 25 child subjects, as its focus was on the treatment of refractory childhood epilepsy. Of these subjects, thirteen were already being treated with the conventional drug Clobazam.

The remaining subjects were used as a control group.

Cannabidiol doses were delivered to the thirteen subjects for a total of eight weeks.

The researchers measured their symptoms and physical responses before the study, at four weeks, and at eight weeks.

Rather remarkably, the results indicated a significant boost to the amount of Clobazam (or CLB) in the bloodstream, as a result of the presence of cannabidiol.

The average increase for the child patients was around 80%. Crucially, nine members of the group demonstrated a

50% reduction in seizure symptoms. Not only that, but the effect was sustained even as the researchers decreased the actual amounts of Clobazam being delivered.

The findings are helpful; because they support the idea that cannabidiol can be used as a supplementary drug to boost the impact of more conventional treatments.

The researchers of this study were, therefore, happy to recommend that cannabidiol be considered a safe and effective medication for refractory childhood epilepsy [107]. As there are many forms of epilepsy which are very difficult to treat, the outcome could be a valuable one.

Cannabidiol Improves Brain and Liver Function in Mice with Acute Organ Failure

The most commonly acknowledged and understood form of liver disease, at least by the general public, is alcohol related organ failure. [108]

This occurs when alcohol addiction causes irreparable damage to the liver. However, there are actually more than a hundred different types of liver disease. Some are caused by lifestyle – being overweight, for example – and others are a result of underlying health conditions like hepatitis. [109]

Either way, liver disease is a big killer in western nations and scientists have spent many years working on viable and effective treatments.

A number have turned their focus to cannabidiol, in a bid to finally determine whether this wonder substance can help patients with organ failure turn their symptoms around. In 2011, the British Journal of Pharmacology published a lab study on encephalic mice treated with cannabidiol.

The objective of the study was to investigate the clear and unambiguous effects of cannabidiol on the brain and liver function of these sick rodents. To do this, female mice were injected with a chemical designed to bring about liver failure.

They were then split into two groups and one was dosed with cannabidiol. The researchers reviewed their neurological and motor functions, before removing the brains and livers for histopathological analysis. Blood samples were also taken and tested.

The researchers found that induced liver failure severely degraded neurological and cognitive functions, but that both of these could be substantially restored in the presence of cannabidiol.

After being dosed with CBD, motor activity improved and the levels of plasma, ammonia, bilirubin, and essential liver enzymes increased.

Also, astrogliosis within the rodent brains was reduced following cannabidiol consumption. Astrogliosis is one of the clearest neurological indications that brain cells are being damaged due to chronic disease. [110]

So, the fact that the rate and severity of the process fell, as a result of cannabidiol treatments, is very important.

While the results of the study cannot be generalized to humans, they do point to a positive contribution from cannabis plant extracts when it comes to reducing the symptoms of liver failure and, perhaps, even reversing them. [111] It is now up to medical scientists to broaden the outcomes and investigate whether they can be extended to humans.

Fear of Public Speaking and Social Interaction Is Reduced with Cannabidiol

This next case study is very interesting, becauseit doesn;t rarely involve degenerative physical or neurological disease. [112] These are the two areas which cannabidiol research seems to have been entirely focused on over the last ten years and there has been little examination of broader, more common social impairments. For instance, Generalized Social Anxiety Disorder (or SAD) is very prevalent within western countries.

This anxiety condition can make it extremely difficult to live a normal life. Meeting new people, interacting with colleagues, and presenting oneself are all tough tasks. [113] Public speaking tends to be a major fear for those with SAD, even though it is a skill that is needed in all kinds of different situations. [114] Tthe condition can impair the ability to get a job, make friends, and form close relationships, the discovery of an effective treatment is a top priority.

The Journal of Neuropsychopharmacology detailed a study, in 2011, which focused on the impact of cannabidiol on society anxiety.

The clinical links between anxiety disorders and cannabidiol are certainly not new. For many years, scientists have been aware of an anxiolytic property of CBD. So, the researchers did expect to discover a positive correlation between the amount of cannabidiol consumed and the degree of anxiety experienced. [115]

The study was a double blind randomized trial. This means that none of the participants were of aware of which group they belonged to; they did not know if they had been given a placebo or a dose of cannabidiol.

They were given the treatment (or a placebo) and asked to perform a simulated public speaking test ninety minutes later.

During the test, their vital signs (heart rate, blood pressure, etc.) were recorded and their mood was assessed two different measures or scales.

The Visual Analogue Mood Scale [116] and the Negative Self-Statement Scale [117] were used to determine mood and level of anxiety. This data was collected at six separate points during the course of the test. The researchers found that a preliminary dose of cannabidiol substantially reduced anxiety, cognitive impairment, and general discomfort while speaking. The treated participants demonstrated much fewer 'alert' signals than the placebo group and appeared to be more relaxed and not 'on guard.' [118]

For the researchers, this was a compelling outcome and clear evidence of the potential use of cannabidiol as an anti-anxiety treatment.

They saw no worrying side effects and they knew that the results couldn't be attributed to bias, because the subjects didn't know if they had been given the cannabidiol. Double blind techniques are particularly important in studies on social responses, because they help researchers prevent subjects from behaving in a way that is unnatural. [119]

Marijuana Compound Prevents Degenerative Eye Problems in Diabetics

In 2006, a research team at the Medical College of Georgia published a series of ground breaking discoveries that link cannabidiol to the treatment of diabetic retinopathy. [120]

The uncovering of such a connection has great value for the medical industry, as degenerative eye problems are a very common symptom of long term diabetes. [121] They are often the kind of symptoms that don't get as much care or attention as they should.

After all, inherited diabetes is one disease made up of many individual issues and strains on the body.

Patients have to be extremely cautious about their general health for the entirety of their lives; regular eye exams, dental inspections, and proper care of the legs and feet are very important. [122] The focus tends to be on treating diabetes via artificial insulin control, in order to control all of its physical symptoms. [123] There is less emphasis on what can be done to mitigate individual problems.

The study is quite different in that respect, but it also represents one of the first suggestions that cannabidiol might have a positive impact on the health of the eye. The study tested a group of male lab rats.

They were first injected with a chemical that is toxic to insulin, as a way to bring about an induced form of diabetes. This was combined with careful and controlled fasting for a period of two weeks. Once the rats were showing signs of diabetic dysfunction, they were split into groups and one group was injected with cannabidiol. [124]

The animals were then humanely sacrificed and their eyes removed for further analysis.

The results showed that, when given cannabidiol, the diabetic rats demonstrated a significantly slower rate of retinal decline. The researchers believe that this is because the compound functions (in several different ways) as a protectant for the blood vessels in the eyes. Diabetic retinopathy is characterized by the development of leaks within these blood vessels, [125] but cannabidiol seems to minimize the damage.

While the researchers couldn't find any evidence to suggest that cannabidiol affects blood glucose, either positively or negatively, the discovery of a link between the compound and the health of the eyes is valuable.

For the researchers at the helm of this study, it means that there is potential for intervention in the development of the condition; crucially, before these leaks in the retina start to appear.

Diabetic retinopathy is currently the leading cause of blindness in adults in the US, so a breakthrough here would be a huge success for the medical industry.

67-Year-Old Female Shrinks Brain Tumor with Cannabidiol

Just recently, in 2016, the case of a 67-year-old female patient diagnosed with a pituitary tumor appeared in the Endocrine Society journal. [126] It provides further strong evidence of a link between cannabidiol and the regression of cancerous cells. It is important to note that the study focused on just this one patient, so its results cannot be generalized to a wider population. However, it is valuable when considered alongside the many other larger trials that have discovered similar findings. [127]

A pituitary macroadenoma is a type of benign tumor of the brain. It is benign because it does not attack the cells as cancerous tumors do. It may be left untreated without putting the life of the patient in danger.

This does not mean, however, that the tumor has no symptoms. As it grows on the pituitary gland, it can wreak havoc with the regulation of hormones. Symptoms include intense headaches, impaired eyesight, dizziness, weight loss, and dysfunction of the sexual organs. [128]

In some cases, it also leads to the development of Cushing's syndrome. This causes unsightly red marks across the thighs, buttocks, stomach, and arms. [129] The 67-year old patient in the study did not have this condition or acromegaly (excessive growth), but she was diagnosed with a pituitary tumor. Following the diagnosis, the growth continued to get bigger and began to interfere with the optic chiasm. [130] She was advised to undergo surgery to mitigate this.

It was at this point that the patient made the independent decision to start taking cannabidiol in an attempt to shrink the tumor. She did this for four months and subsequent tests revealed that the growth had indeed been reduced in size.

This made it easier and safer for surgeons to remove the tumor.

Six weeks after surgery, additional tests showed that levels of urinary free cortisol and salivary cortisol had begun to return to a healthy state.

The patient continues to recover well and take regular doses of cannabidiol.

The study is an interesting one for a number of reasons. One reason being, cannabidiol, when it is tested in a medical capacity, tends to be tested on aggressive forms of cancer. [131] Researchers have discovered remarkable findings in this area and there is much evidence to believe that the plant extract could be a very successful anti-cancer treatment. Yet, it also has promise as a hormone regulator. It reduces pituitary hormone levels and brings cortisol back to a healthy state, even if the function of the pituitary gland has been compromised. [132]

Cannabidiol Treatments Represent a Breakthrough in Myocarditis Research

While there are all kinds of different cardiovascular diseases and dysfunctions, myocarditis is one of the hardest to understand. [133] It is a disease that is characterized by extreme inflammation and degradation of the muscle in the heart. The problem is that it tends to develop very quickly and lead to death without much warning. Even more unsettling is the fact that myocarditis is most prevalent in young adults, who are otherwise very healthy.

According to statistics, around 5-20% of all sudden deaths in young adults can be attributed to myocarditis.

It can be brought on by a number of different things; viral infections, autoimmune disorders, exposure to environmental toxins, and adverse responses to new medications. It kills by bringing about total heart failure, so scientists are very keen to discover effective treatments. [134] Once such team of researchers carried out a study on the relationship between cannabidiol and myocarditis.

The study involved tests on lab rodents.

Autoimmune myocarditis was artificially induced, in order to bring about T cell mediated inflammation, progressive death of the cardiomyocyte cells, and other forms of cardiovascular dysfunction.

After being treated with cannabidiol, however, the mice demonstrated a less intense inflammatory response and a slower rate of deterioration. Cardiovascular dysfunction decreased and so did myocardial fibrosis.

The results suggest that cannabidiol could be used as a successful treatment for those already diagnosed with autoimmune myocarditis and a number of other related autoimmune disorders.

In addition to this, due to the fact that the compound can help regulate how the immune system responds to changes within the body, it may have a positive impact on organ transplantation and the likelihood of acceptance. [135] This is an important breakthrough, because many of the existing treatments for myocarditis are either ineffective or they produce severe side effects and toxicities within the body. [136]

Cannabidiol Increases Urge to Swim and Survive in Lab Rodents

[137] For many years, scientists conducting studies on possible anti-depression treatments have used a controversial test called the 'forced swim test'. [138] This evaluates the strength of a compulsion to survive by placing mice in a tank of water. If they swim, they are judged to be fighting for survival and, therefore, be demonstrating a healthy instinct for self-preservation. If they refuse to swim or move sluggishly, this instinct is thought to be impaired. [139]

The test is important, because the instinct to 'save oneself' is often absent in people who are clinically depressed. Like the mice, they are unlikely to fight for their own survival and, if placed in a similar situation, may simply let dangerous circumstances affect them. [140] Regardless of the moral status of the study – which has been questioned by animal rights campaigners – it remains a popular test and it is routinely used to evaluate the efficacy of treatments for anxiety and mood disorders. [141]

In 2009, a team of researchers used the test to determine the presence of a link between cannabidiol and the treatment of depressive tendencies.

They took a number of mice and split them into two groups. One of the groups was dosed with cannabidiol. All of the mice were then placed in tanks of water and their behaviors recorded.

A number of the animals were also placed in an open field test to ascertain their degree of interest and awareness.

After a dose of 30mg of cannabidiol, the mice displayed significantly more physical activity and motion while in the tanks.

This effect was further investigated by giving some of the animals another treatment designed to block the cannabis plant extract.

Once mitigated, the mice returned to a state of reduced activity just like the ones that hadn't been dosed with cannabidiol before the swim test.

The results of the open field test showed no significant changes. The mice were not any more willing to explore after consuming cannabidiol.

However, the researchers believe that the boost in mobility for the CBD mice was due to its antidepressant like effects. They compare this to imipramine, which is a common pharmaceutical intervention for depression. [142] According to their conclusions, the power of cannabidiol is likely explained by its ability to activate or 'switch on' the 5-HT1A receptors.

Treating Diabetic Mice with Cannabidiol Alleviates Their Symptoms

Diabetes is one of the most dangerous chronic and degenerative diseases that we know of. [143] While it may not kill as fast as cancer, it is highly debilitating and causes millions of deaths every year in western nations. [144] For this reason alone, it has been the subject of fierce interest from medical scientists for many years. Most of the big pharmaceutical companies are desperate to become the first provider of a 'cure' for this disease. [145]

Thus far, much of the clinical testing has been carried out on lab mice.

A 2008 study used a sample of NOD (non-obese diabetes prone) female rodents to investigate the impact of cannabidiol treatments on diabetes symptoms.

The results are rather fascinating, because they suggest that cannabidiol is a great way to slow down the progression of dysfunctions associated with chronic and late stage diabetes.

The researchers dosed 11-14 week old NOD mice with cannabidiol. All of the rodents were either in an early or an established phase of the disease. When tested again, only 32% of the dosed mice showed any symptoms at all. This rose to a staggering 86-100% of the mice that were not treated with the compound first. They also recorded a significant drop in inflammatory cytokines, which work as a kind of emergency defense system for the body and cause a variety of dysfunctions. [146]

Also, the pancreatic functions of the CBD treated mice were noticeably healthier. This is a valuable finding, because the pancreas produces insulin. The more islet cells that are contained within the pancreas, the more efficiently it can regulate insulin production. [147] The mice treated with cannabidiol had more islets than the control group. As such, the researchers concluded that cannabidiol is a safe and effective treatment for Type 1 diabetes in humans.

Type 1 diabetes has long proved a challenge for clinicians and doctors. Unlike Type 2 diabetes, it cannot be controlled through diet alone and patients must stick to a regular daily schedule of insulin injections and blood measurement procedures. As the disease is genetic, rather than related to lifestyle, the main focus has been on early detection and education. However, cannabidiol is currently proving to be a very promising source of potential treatment. [148]

Study Shows That Isolating Cannabidiol from Cannabis Sativa Allows It to Become a Cancer Killer

[149] For a long time, there has been debate over not just whether cannabis really does have a positive impact on physical and neurological health, but also whether this can be attributed to the whole plant or just part of it. Certainly for critics of cannabis legalization, the idea that THC might be as beneficial as cannabidiol (which is non-psychotropic) has always been a challenging one. It is a question that scientists have been interested in as well. [150]

A 2016 study on cancer research and potential treatments sought to find an answer.

It isolated cannabidiol from the rest of the plant and tested it against a cannabis sativa crude extract.

The aim was to determine the impact of both when introduced to human cervical cancer cells. The results of the study showed that cannabidiol is an extremely powerful substance; perhaps a lot more powerful than we acknowledge it to potentially be.

It was able to stop the cancerous cells from multiplying and it induced cell apoptosis in all tests.

This is a type of programmed cell death that results in the cancerous tissues being starved of the things that they need to survive. [151] So, in short, the cannabidiol cannot directly eradicate cancer cells, but it does have the ability to make their environment more hostile. After interacting with the cannabidiol, the samples demonstrated an overexpression of caspase and P53. [152]

These are two chemicals that are involved in immune responses. Their increased presence leads to a faster deterioration of cancerous tissues. [153] The researchers discovered that it is the cannabidiol, specifically, which brings about these changes rather than the cannabis plant as a whole.

This is a useful finding for a number of reasons. The first is that it shows CBD has great potential as a cancer treatment. The second is that it is possible to pursue cannabidiol as a treatment option, without the need to incorporate or tolerate the presence of THC.

As there are scores of families, all around the world, who have been using cannabidiol to treat their children for years, it is in the best interests of the pharmaceutical industry to come up with a safe and approved formula.

The compound has produced remarkable results for minors suffering with severe epilepsy, yet parents are still fighting to have their treatments recognized simply because the extract is wrongly associated with THC and recreational smoking. [154]

Could Cannabidiol Be Used to Make General Anesthetics Safer?

One area of research that rarely receives much attention is the relationship between plant based compounds and anesthesia. This may be simply because the clinical urgency surrounding it is just not as intense as, say, cancer treatments or epilepsy medications. Yet, scientific research on anesthesia is extremely valuable. Every year, studies are conducted which make general anesthetics safer for patients. [156]

This is the main goal, of course. No matter how routine the procedure, putting somebody to 'sleep' comes with all kinds of hidden dangers.

There is no way to know for sure how a person will react to an anesthetic, so experts are keen to find safer alternatives or ways to sedate patients with smaller amounts of sedative gas or pharmaceuticals. [157] This was partly the aim of a 1974 study, which was republished by the British Journal of Pharmacology in 2012.

The study looked at the relationship between cannabidiol and the effects of common anesthetics.

The anesthetics used were pentobarbitone and ether and mice were the test subjects. When dosed with a cannabidiol compound, the duration of the pentobarbitone anesthetic was substantially extended. The greatest effect was seen if the mice were dosed with CBD anywhere between twenty minutes to two hours beforehand.

A difference could still be observed if the mice were dosed right up to eight hours before being given the pentobarbitone, but at this distance from the anesthetic, the impact was smaller. The duration of the anesthetic was maximally prolonged when doses were given no longer than two hours prior to the anesthetic.

On the other hand, the ether anesthetic was not changed by the presence of cannabidiol.

The researchers concluded that combining cannabis extracts with pentobarbitone could, potentially, result in an ability to reduce the amount of pharmaceuticals used in surgical interventions.

If cannabidiol can make a smaller amount of an anesthetic last for a longer time, surgeons may be able to administer reduced quantities. This is particularly helpful for older patients, young children, babies, and anybody with underlying health issues that might be affected by the delivery of general anesthetics. [158]

Can Cannabidiol Help Humans Learn When and Why to Fear?

One of the most interesting studies on the neurological impact of cannabidiol was first published in 2013. [159] At the time, it was the only study ever to assess the relationship between CBD and extinction learning in human beings. For this reason, its results were always going to be ground breaking and of great value to cognitive science.

Up until this point, only mice had been evaluated in a similar manner.

Extinction learning is a very complex process of social conditioning. It describes the way in which a human (or an animal) learns how to adapt to perceived threats. [160] For example, if a person were to walk across an extremely high bridge for the first time, they might feel frightened. They would exhibit classic fear responses like a faster heart rate, clammy skin, and a slight tremor.

However, if they had to walk over this same bridge every single day, without incident, the likelihood is that they'd stop being afraid.

This is a product of extinction learning; the ability to adapt to familiar environments and situations. It would be no use to the person to continue being scared. In fact, it would actually make their life more difficult, so the fear stops becoming an automatic response.

The height is still dangerous and does pose a risk, but behaving in the right way is enough to eliminate it. This is a very simple example and extinction learning is a much more complex phenomenon that influences daily life in a thousand different ways. [161]

To study its relationship to cannabidiol, which has long been touted as a substance with anti-anxiety properties, [162] the researchers hooked up human volunteers to a box that administered mild electric shocks.

They were not aware of when the box would shock and when it would not. Naturally, their attempts to anticipate the shocks led to a series of physiological anxiety and fear responses. After a time, all of the subjects (including the control not dosed with CBD) began to lose their fear, because they knew what was coming.

Interestingly though, the researchers found that this response was noticeably greater in the subjects given cannabidiol.

They lost their fear faster and demonstrated less intense physiological fear responses. It was concluded that cannabidiol could, potentially, be used as a treatment for anxiety disorders. Extreme anxiety, in many ways, is just an overexpression of a natural fear response, so CBD might be able to soothe it and provide an effective treatment. [163]

Cannabidiol Protects the Brain from the Damage Caused By Excess Iron

[164] Over the years, there have been a number of high profile studies linking excessive brain iron to the development of neurological disorders like Parkinson's and Alzheimer's. [165] In 2014, the journal of Molecular Neurobiology published a study on the impact of cannabidiol consumption and levels of harmful brain iron. It represents a vital step forward on the road to discovering effective, safe treatments for these neurodegenerative conditions.

The study closely observed the expression of brain proteins in a number of rodent subjects suffering from neurodegenerative disease.

The focus was not just on how much iron was accumulated in the brain, but also on the rate of apoptosis and specific DNA fragmentation. Apoptosis can be a positive process if it is occurring within harmful cells (such as cancerous tissues), but it poses a great threat to brain function if the wrong cells are being targeted for destruction. [166]

The researchers discovered that rats dosed with cannabidiol demonstrated smaller amounts of accumulated iron, as well as healthier levels of hippocampal DNM1L, caspase 3, and synaptophysin. [167] If dosed in the right way, these levels began to more closely resemble the healthy control group. The results suggest that cannabidiol is an effective memory rescuing, neuroprotective substance which can regulate brain iron and preserve brain function.

This has huge consequences for Alzheimer's and Parkinson's patients, for whom brain cell death leads to a severely impaired memory and, often, an inability to recall even simple tasks or processes. The researchers, therefore, concluded that cannabidiol should be considered as a potential neuroprotective treatment. [168]

What Does the Future Hold for Cannabidiol Research and Investigation?

It is not easy to predict where the course of cannabidiol research and clinical investigation will end up.

While it is pretty much certain that the number of studies and the amount of interest will significantly increase, over the coming years, the existing barriers to its exploration remain a problem.

The FDA is very clear on the fact that, if cannabidiol does become an approved medical and therapeutic treatment, it will be as the isolated compound and not as part of the whole cannabis plant. [169]

The reasons behind this have already been discussed in great detail, but it is worth acknowledging how much an obstacle this could be for researchers.

The social stigma surrounding cannabis won't be eased any time soon if regulators are too afraid to allow even licensed clinicians and medical experts to scrutinize it. And, if the cannabis plant continues to be the subject of misinformation and misconception for the general public, cannabidiol will too.

This is not to mention the fact that other parts of the plant have, themselves, been linked to medical and therapeutic benefits.

According to scientists, the future of the compound needs to be all about transparency and data sharing. Research must be made publically available, rather than being hidden away, and those working on it need to be more willing to collaborate. [170] There is every chance that, given enough funding and support, they could one day produce a cannabidiol based cure for a big killer like cancer.

Which Cannabidiol Products Are Approved and Trusted By the Market?

For those who are keen to integrate cannabidiol into their own lives and routines, there are many choices. This can be both a good and a bad thing, because it means that picking reliable products is tough sometimes.

Availability will depend entirely on how a particular state or region regulates the sale of cannabidiol. This will also determine price, quality, and the varieties offered from individual vendors.

To make sure that reliable, safe products are used, it is necessary to carry out personal research and make personal judgements regarding the suitability of cannabidiol for certain types of lifestyles, medical statuss, and states of health. At the moment, consumers are very much on their own when it comes to the use of this wonderful substance.

They can consult medical studies and read up on the many success stories from around the world, but the reality is that cannabidiol is not yet an officially endorsed treatment.

Therefore, taking it is a personal decision. It is possible though – and strongly advised – that those planning to treat a medical condition with cannabidiol speak with a doctor first.

It is an herbal extract and allergies to plant based compounds are common. Having that clinical support is important, just in case an adverse reaction is experienced.

This is extremely unlikely, but all therapeutic and pharmaceutical treatments come with some risk, because every patient responds differently to these induced physiological changes.

Tips for Buying the Best Cannabidiol Oils and Tinctures

It is important to be aware that the term 'oil,' in this context can refer to a number of different products. Essentially though, cannabidiol oil should be sold in small amounts (usually in clear glass bottles) and have an easy to use applicator.

This could be a small dropper nozzle or a spray function. Cannabidiol is used in conjunction with vape pens and larger vaporizer devices, but it can also be ingested directly, without the need for any other kind of apparatus.

The three most important things to think about when buying cannabidiol oil are concentration, purity, and source.

Concentration is the first decision that should be made, because it determines how intense an effect the substance will have. [171] To reiterate, cannabidiol cannot produce a high in the conventional sense, but it will make a person feel sleepy in large amounts. To avoid this, opt for a low concentration blend or formula. [172]

When cannabidiol oil is taken to relieve chronic pain, sometimes, the drowsiness is a worthwhile compromise.

However, this depends on all kinds of different factors; what time of day it is being taken, type of occupation, lifestyle, and the presence of other pharmaceutical medications. [173] Generally, these products range in concentration strength from 0.1 to 0.26%. Keep this in mind when browsing and remember that starting small is usually a better idea than jumping in head first with a super strength oil.

Purity is another important factor; though personal judgement is advised.

For most users, it is really important to buy from organic and all natural vendors as, being a plant product; there is a chance that non-organic oils have come into contact with pesticides. [174] There is a distinct lack of research on the differences between organic and non-organic cannabidiol, so first timer buyers are encouraged to make the choice that they feel most comfortable with.

It is worth pointing out that organic producers are the ones most willing to list every step of the production process.

Many of these vendors give their customers enough information to follow the manufacturing stages right back from bottling to seed.

Like most herbal supplements, cannabidiol can be very cheap or very expensive. The better the quality and purity, the higher the price will be, though it is possible to pick up quality mid-range oils as well.

Knowing What to Look Out for When Choosing Hemp Seed Products

If a cannabidiol oil or tincture doesn't appeal, there are alternative ways to consume it.

One of the most wholesome is in the form of hulled hemp seeds.

They are extremely diverse, because they can be eaten raw, cooked, crushed, toasted, or prepared in a plethora of other ways.

To make sure that the product being purchased is of a high quality, check where the seeds have been produced before buying.

Interestingly, Canada is often cited as the country which produces the tastiest hemp seeds in the world.

This can be attributed to the fact that Canadian producers have to adhere to strict laws and regulations set out by the government.

For instance, they can only sell or use hemp seed varieties that are included on the list of Approved Cultivars. [175] All varieties are free of genetic modification. Also, Canadian farmers are not allowed to use pesticides when growing and farming hemp. [176]

There are other producers, in other nations, but none offer products as stringently verified and scrutinized as Canadian hemp seeds.

The flavor should be pleasant, with a slightly nutty taste similar to sunflower seeds.

However, hemp seeds are noticeably softer.

Do be cautious and informed when buying because there are many subpar products on the market as well.

Learning How to Use Hemp Protein Powders in the Right Way

Hemp (or CBD) protein powders can be a really valuable dietary supplement, especially for people who like to hit the gym. [177] It should be noted, however, that it is lower in protein than some of the more conventional options like whey powder.

For standard protein needs though, it is an effective addition to an active lifestyle.

It can also be safely combined with other organic powders like pea and rice products, as a way to boost its muscle supporting capacities. [178] Some more expensive varieties, offer a 'hemp protein concentrate' which is higher in protein, but lower in omega fatty acids.

Either product can be effective, depending on what the user is hoping to achieve. [179] Always buy from reputable vendors that are happy to disclose information about how the powder was manufactured.

Advice on Shopping for the Highest Quality Vape Pens and Oils

The meteoric rise of vape pens has seen the introduction of cannabidiol vape oil.

This is one of the most common ways to consume the plant extract, primarily because it already feels familiar to most people.

It is easy to do, the products are simple to source, and using them in public is still quite a discreet process.

The downside to the popularity of cannabidiol vape oils is that there's now so many of them on the market.

It can be tough, particularly for new users, to know where to start when looking for high quality products.

However, there are a few basic rules that can make the process less intimidating.

The first thing to think about is whether you're happy to invest in flavored oils.

This can be a controversial subject among connoisseurs, with some people being quite fond of the juicy varieties and others firmly believing that no additives should ever be used.

To ensure that a cannabidiol vape oil is organic, the only practical option is to pick up an unflavored product.

Unaltered oils contain no extra chemicals or artificial substances and are, as such, considered to be at the higher end of the market. In addition, check websites for certificates of analysis and purity.

This is a good indication that the cannabidiol has been produced and manufactured to very precise, high standards.

Final Thoughts on the Regulation, Distribution, and Use of Cannabidiol

What Does the FDA Think about Cannabidiol Being Used as a Medicine?

It is clear that the FDA is very aware of how widespread the use of cannabidiol is, particularly as a medicinal and therapeutic treatment.

Nevertheless, it has yet to officially endorse or approve any product containing the compound.

It is quick to stress this when asked about its opinion on the scientific merits of CBD oils and other forms.

It does not, from a general perspective, consider its use to be criminal, but state authorities have the final word on this.

Why Hasn't the FDA Approved Cannabidiol Treatments Yet?

At the moment, the current answer to this is that the FDA does not know for sure if cannabidiol is safe to use as a medical or therapeutic treatment.

This is in direct conflict with the many people around the world who continue to consume it without side effects.

It does claim to be in supportive of approved, licensed medical research on its therapeutic potential.

Could Parents Who Give Their Children Cannabidiol Face Legal Penalties?

Once again, this depends entirely on the state and the nature of its rules and regulations. The FDA does not have jurisdiction in this regard.

It cannot and has not acknowledged the belief that cannabidiol can be a safe treatment for childhood epilepsy and other conditions.

It stresses that parents should only ever use pharmaceuticals that it has thoroughly tested and approved.

It makes no comment on the many cases of parents giving their children a renewed quality of life via cannabidiol dosages and treatments.

Does the FDA Have Evidence That Cannabidiol Can Be Harmful to the Health?

The FDA received a negligible amount of reports detailing adverse effects of cannabidiol usage, primarily because it only deals with approved and endorsed products.

It advises those interested in finding out more to consult medical trials and studies. Interestingly, this is quite a positive experience for most.

The negative reports are certainly outweighed by the positive ones, no matter where on the internet research is being conducted.

Is It Possible to Fail a Routine Drugs Test After Medicating with Cannabidiol?

It is highly unlikely that this would happen, as cannabidiol is not the same as THC and this is what mandatory drugs tests are looking for.

The only small chance that it could be picked up is if a variety with a slightly higher amount of THC has been consumed.

Once again, this is quite unlikely, because reputable cannabidiol vendors don't sell products containing anything but trace amounts of THC.

In addition to this, using the substance is not illegal.

It cannot produce a high and has no debilitating impact on the brain.

Can Cannabidiol Interfere with Other Prescribed Medications?

There is always a very small chance that consuming cannabidiol could cause other medications to be less effective.

It is important to be fully aware of this.

It is not a serious problem and doctors also advise patients not to consume things like grapefruit, for example, shortly before taking pills.

There is plenty of information online, so it is easy to check how different drugs and treatments respond to cannabidiol before deciding to take it.

Can You Consume Cannabidiol Incorrectly and Are There Any Risks?

It is perfectly possible to consume cannabidiol inefficiently and to, therefore, not get the maximum benefit. There is no risk involved though.

All that will happen is that the impact won't be as powerful as expected.

If too much is ingested, there may be an intense feeling of tiredness, but no side effects any worse than this have been identified.

For a first time user, the recommendation is to be relaxed and somewhere comfortable.

It is a really good idea to avoid things like driving just in case the drowsiness is a little stronger than predicted.

Has Anybody Ever Died Due to the Use of Cannabidiol?

At this point, there has never been a single instance of a person dying or developing any kind of illness because they have consumed cannabidiol, even on a regular basis.

It simply hasn't ever happened and any claims that it has are, fortunately, false.

While the medical industry is still playing catch up when it comes to cannabidiol, even its critics cannot produce any convincing evidence that it is unsafe for use.

Why the Story of the 'Miracle Compound' Will Only Get More Fascinating

As discussed, there is really only one direction for the development of cannabidiol to move in. In many ways, the transition towards full approval has already begun, though regulatory bodies like the FDA are reluctant to acknowledge it.

For once though, it is the people – the general public – who will lead the charge.

Many of them have already defined local and state laws to gain access to cannabidiol and other cannabis plant extracts, because they know that the legal risks outweigh the potential health benefits.

It is their accounts that tell the real story of cannabidiol and its many, many neurological and physiological uses. This is why it is important for their voices to be heard, among the cold, hard facts produced by the medical community.

Both sides form an essential part of the story and it is only when both are considered together that a full and comprehensive picture will emerge.

CBD Vendor List

In non-partial alphabetical order.

CBD Essence - http://cannabiscbdoil.org/cbd-essence

Charlotte's Web - http://cannabiscbdoil.org/charlottes-web

Elixinol - http://cannabiscbdoil.org/elixinol

Endoca - http://cannabiscbdoil.org/endoca

VapeBright - http://cannabiscbdoil.org/vapebright

References

[1] Brooks, Megan (September 1, 2016) 'More US Adults Using Marijuana as Attitudes Change' http://www.medscape.com/viewarticle/868282

[2] Becker, Sam (May 22, 2015) '10 Countries Leading the Push for Marijuana Legalisation' http://www.cheatsheet.com/politics/10-countries-that-have-or-will-see-marijuana-legalization.html/?a=viewall

[3] Pop Pot (April 15, 2015) 'CBD Not Same as Medical Marijuana' http://www.poppot.org/2015/04/15/cannabidiol-or-cbd-is-not-same-as-medical-marijuana/

[4] Genece, Clifford (February 10, 2016). 'CBD: 13 Commonly Asked Questions' https://www.honeycolony.com/article/13-common-questions-about-cbd/

[5] Leaf Science (March 16, 2014) '6 Surprising Facts about THC' http://www.leafscience.com/2014/03/16/6-surprising-facts-thc/

[6] Mary Jane's Diary (August 18, 2016) 'CBD: Cures Cancer, Won't Get You High' http://maryjanesdiary.com/cannabidiol-cbd/

[7] Freeman, Makia (June 8, 2016) 'CBD: The Cat is Out of the Bag with this Natural Cure All' http://wakeup-world.com/2016/07/08/cannabidiol-cbd-the-cats-out-of-the-bag-with-this-natural-cure-all/

[8] Rucke, Katie (July 15, 2014) 'Hemp Oil versus CBD Oil: What Is the Difference?' http://www.mintpressnews.com/hemp-oil-versus-cbd-oil-whats-the-difference/193962/

[9] McElrath KJ (July 15, 2015) 'Medical Marijuana Could Be a Medical Cure for So Many' http://trofire.com/2015/07/16/medical-marijuana-could-be-a-miracle-cure-for-so-many-yet-big-pharma-is-trying-to-stop-it/

[10] Dorm, Drake (Retrieved October 6, 2016) 'CBD May Help Treat Anxiety Disorder' https://www.medicaljane.com/2014/05/28/study-cannabidiol-cbd-may-help-treat-social-anxiety-disorder/

[11] Walia, Arjun (August 23, 2013) '20 Medical Studies That Show Cannabis Can Be a Potential Cure for Cancer' http://www.collective-evolution.com/2013/08/23/20-medical-studies-that-prove-cannabis-can-cure-cancer/

[12] Lee, Martin (March 4, 2014) 'CBD: The Marijuana Miracle' https://www.projectcbd.org/article/cbd-marijuana-miracle

[13] Weed Geek (November 18th, 2013) '12 Medical Marijuana Miracles You Should Know About' http://www.weed-geek.com/12-medical-marijuana-miracles-you-should-know-about/

[14] Torres, Marco (May 12, 2014) '5 Disease Proven to Respond Better to Cannabis'

http://preventdisease.com/news/14/051214_5-Diseases-Proven-To-Respond-Better-To-Cannabis-Than-Prescription-Drugs.shtml

[15] Supplement Police (Retrieved October 6, 2016) 'CBD Rich Hemp Oil' https://supplementpolice.com/cbd-oil/

[16] Terps, Tyler (November 3, 2015) '10 Little Known Uses for CBD' http://hightimes.com/culture/10-little-known-uses-for-cbd/

[17] Gerard, Arielle (Retrieved October 6, 2016) 'CBD in the Management of Schizophrenia' https://www.medicaljane.com/2015/03/02/systematic-review/

[18] MacGill, Markus (October 13, 2013) 'Chemicals in Marijuana Protect Nervous System against MS' http://www.medicalnewstoday.com/articles/267161.php

[19] The Global Diabetes Community (Retrieved October 5, 2016) 'Cannabis and Diabetes' http://www.diabetes.co.uk/recreational-drugs/cannabis.html

[20] Sander, Jason (July 23, 2016) 'Can Cannabis Help Treat Sleep Disorders?' https://www.marijuanatimes.org/can-cannabis-help-treat-sleep-disorders/

[21] Truth on Pot (September 24, 2014) '5 Differences between CBD and THC' http://www.truthonpot.com/2014/09/24/5-differences-between-cbd-vs-thc/

[22] Endoca (May 16, 2016) 'CBD Oil Children: Cannabis Makes a Difference' https://www.endoca.com/blog/news/parents-seek-cbd-oil-children/

[23] Medithrive (Retrieved October 6, 2016). 'How to Use CBD Oil' http://medithrive.com/how-to-use-cbd-oil/

[24] Organic Cosmos (Retrieved October 5, 2016) 'Safety and Dosage'
http://organiccosmos.com/safety-and-dosage/

[25] The Chill Bud (Retrieved October 6, 2016) 'Understanding the Different Types of Cannabis Oil'
http://thechillbud.com/understanding-the-different-types-of-cannabis-oil-and-how-theyre-made/

[26] Rabinski, Gooey (October 5, 2015) 'What is a Cannabis Tincture?'
https://www.whaxy.com/learn/what-is-cannabis-tincture

[27] Maurer, Leah (March 10, 2011) 'The Most Underrated of All Marijuana Products'
https://www.theweedblog.com/the-most-underrated-of-all-marijuana-products-weed-tinctures/

[28] Hadfield, Pamela (July 3, 2015) 'How Medical Marijuana Tinctures Helped Melt Away My Anxiety and Stress'
https://www.hellomd.com/health-wellness/how-medical-marijuana-tinctures-helped-melt-away-my-anxiety-and-stress

[29] News Medical (Retrieved October 5, 2016) ‘What is a Liposome?’ http://www.news-medical.net/life-sciences/What-is-a-Liposome.aspx

[30] Global News Wire (May 5, 2016) ‘Elixonal Introduces the X-Pen’

[31] One Green Planet (Retrieved October 6, 2016) ‘5 Things to Do with Hemp Protein Powder’ http://www.onegreenplanet.org/vegan-food/things-to-do-with-hemp-protein-powder-you-havent-tried-yet/

[32] Harris, Kimi (Match 11, 2009) ‘Hemp Seed: Nutritional Values and Thoughts’ http://www.thenourishinggourmet.com/2009/03/hemp-seed-nutritional-value-and-thoughts.html

[33] Chaey, Christina (May 11, 2015) ‘Everything You Need to Know about Eating Hemp Seeds’

http://www.bonappetit.com/test-kitchen/ingredients/article/hemp-seeds

[34] Ponds, Amielia (December 9, 2009) 'Hemp Protein: Eat the Nutrients' http://www.naturalnews.com/027691_hemp_protein_seeds.html

[35] Davis, Allison (February 23, 2015) 'Can You Get a High from Marijuana Lip Balm?' http://nymag.com/thecut/2015/02/will-this-lip-balm-get-you-high.html

36. Endoca (July 4, 2016). 'Slow Pace of Scientific Validation for CBD' https://www.endoca.com/blog/news/cbd-scientific-research/

37. Porter, Nanette (Retrieved October 7, 2016) 'Meet the Woman Who Beat Her Lung Cancer with Cannabis Oil.' https://www.medicaljane.com/2015/06/11/meet-the-woman-who-beat-her-lung-cancer- with-cannabis-oil/

38. Chris Beat Cancer (Retrieved October 7, 2016) 'Why Your Body's PH Matters'
http://www.chrisbeatcancer.com/alkalize-it-or-why-your-bodys-ph-matters/

39. Suzanne (January 3, 2014). 'Autism/CBD Oil Success Stories'

http://cbdoil.blogspot.co.uk/2014/01/autismcbd-oil-success-stories-joshua.html

40. Wuest, Martin (February 17, 2015) 'What Happened When They Treated Autistic Children with Medical Cannabis'
http://www.collective-evolution.com/2015/02/17/what-happened-when-they-treated-autistic-children-with-medical-cannabis/

41. Canorml (Retrieved October 7, 2016) 'California NORML Patient's Guide to Medical Marijuana'
http://www.canorml.org/medical-marijuana/patients-guide-to-california-law

42. The Journal of Clinical Investigation (October 13, 2005) 'Cannabinoids Promote Embryonic Adult Hippocampus Neurogenesis' https://www.ncbi.nlm.nih.gov/pmc/articles/PMC1253627/

43. Endoca (June 2, 2016). 'Would You Give Your Child CBD Oil?' https://www.endoca.com/blog/discovery/cbd-oil-safe-treatment-babies-children/

44. Liebermann, Oren (May 16, 2016). 'Medical Marijuana for Babies and Their Desperate Parents' http://edition.cnn.com/2016/05/16/health/medical-marijuana-babies/

45. YNetNews (March 27, 2016) 'Medical Marijuana Takes Off in Israel' http://www.ynetnews.com/articles/0,7340,L-4783899,00.html

46. Kloosterman, Karin (March 29, 2012) 'Israeli Medicine Goes to Pot' http://www.israel21c.org/israeli-medicine-goes-to-pot/

47. Second Opinion Group (Retrieved October 7, 2016). 'Our Doctors'
http://www.secondopiniongroup.com/urikramer

48. Endoca (September 12, 2016). 'Nate Diaz Uses CBD Oil As a Neuro-Protectant'
https://www.endoca.com/blog/news/nate-diaz-ufc-competitor-uses-cbd-oil-neuroprotectant/

49. BBC News (October 6, 2016). 'Nate Diaz Accepts Anti-Doping Warning'
http://www.bbc.co.uk/sport/37573519

50. Google Webpage/Patents (Retrieved 7 October, 2016) ' Cannabinoids as Antioxidants and Neuro-Protectants'
https://www.google.com/patents/US6630507

51. The University of Nottingham (December 3, 2013) 'Compounds in Cannabis Could Limit Stroke Damage'
https://www.nottingham.ac.uk/news/pressreleases/2013/december/compounds-in-cannabis-could-limit-stroke-damage.aspx

[52] Hello MD (April 19, 2016). 'Treating My Autoimmune Disease with Cannabis Oil' https://www.hellomd.com/health-wellness/constance-finley-s-story-treating-my-autoimmune-disease-with-cannabis-oil

[53] Constance Therapeutics (Retrieved October 10, 2016) 'Constance Finley's Story' http://constancetherapeutics.com/about/constance-finley-bio.html

[54] Yahoo (November 19, 2014). 'Constance Pure Botanical Extracts to Be Guest Speaker at South by Southwest' http://finance.yahoo.com/news/constance-pure-botanical-extracts-medical-211355679.html

[55] Dorm, Drake (Retrieved October 9, 2016). 'Cannabis Oil Continues to Save Lives in the US' https://www.medicaljane.com/2013/11/09/success-stories-cannabis-oil-in-the-us/

[56] Horsley, Lincoln (October 8, 2014) 'Beating Liver Cancer with Cannabis Oil'

http://www.cureyourowncancer.org/michael-cutlers-story-beating-liver-cancer-with-cannabis-oil.html

[57] Hodgekiss, Anna (July 21, 2014) 'Grandfather Claims He Cured His Cancer with Cannabis Oil' http://www.dailymail.co.uk/health/article-2699875/I-cured-cancer-CANNABIS-OIL.html

[58] Simpson, Rick (March 7, 2008) 'How Cannabis Cures Cancer and Why Nobody Knows' http://www.cannabisculture.com/content/2008/03/07/5169

[59] The Health Cure (October 8, 2014) 'Grandfather Claims He Cured His Cancer Breaking Bad Style' http://www.thehealthcure.org/grandfather-63-claims-he-cured-his-cancer-with-breaking-bad-style-homemade-cannabis-oil/

[60] Withnall, Adam (July 14, 2014) 'New Study Reveals Important Details of Marijuana's Anti-Cancer Properties' http://www.independent.co.uk/life-style/health-and-families/health-news/scientists-reveal-how-thc-found-in-cannabis-could-slow-cancer-tumor-growth-9605219.html

[61] Fassa, Paul (December 9, 2014) 'Lung Cancer Patient Miraculously Cured By Cannabis Oil'
http://www.naturalnews.com/047924_lung_cancer_cannabis_oil_medical_marijuana.html

[62] Caregivers for Life (May 6, 2015) 'Cannabis Oil Success Stories'
http://caregiversforlife.net/cannabis-oil-success-stories/?ao_confirm

[63] Care Center (July 2, 2013) 'Does Sugar Feed Cancer?'
http://www.cancercenter.com/discussions/blog/does-sugar-feed-cancer/

[64] Farley, Tim (November 30, 2015) THC Oil Significantly Reduces Seizures among Child Epilepsy Patients'
http://www.reddirtreport.com/red-dirt-news/success-stories-prove-cannabis-thc-oil-significantly-reduce-seizures-among-child

[65] Hope, Heather (May 31, 2015) 'Oklahomans Rally for Medical Marijuana Initiative'
http://www.news9.com/story/29198917/oklahomans-rally-for-medical-marijuana-initiative

[66] Agorist, Matt (June 28, 2015) 'Since Oklahoma Legalised Cannabis Oil'
http://www.alternet.org/oklahoma-legalized-cannabis-oil-these-two-children-have-been-seizure-free-0

[67] Porter, Nanette (Retrieved October 11, 2016) 'Family with Suffering Children Says Cannabis Oil Needs to Be Legal'
https://www.medicaljane.com/2015/06/11/family-with-suffering-children-says-cannabis-oil-treatment-needs-to-be-legal/

[68] Burke, Darla (February 9, 2016) 'Metachromatic Leukodystrophy'
http://www.healthline.com/health/metachromatic-leukodystrophy

[69] Beattie, Jilly (February 12, 2016) 'Illegal Cannabis Oil Stops Terminally Ill Dad's Brain Tumor'

http://www.mirror.co.uk/news/uk-news/illegal-cannabis-oil-stops-terminally-7354970

[70] Moore, Charles (October 23, 2015) 'Cannabis Derived Sativex for MS Spasticity Is Effective and Safe' https://multiplesclerosisnewstoday.com/2015/10/23/cannabis-derived-sativex-ms-related-spasticity-reported-effective-safe/

[71] Morris, Nigel (February 11, 2016) 'Nick Clegg Backs Campaign Calling for Medical Use of Drug' http://www.independent.co.uk/news/uk/politics/cannabis-legalisation-nick-clegg-backs-campaign-calling-for-medical-use-of-drug-a6866271.html

[72] Young, Sandra (August 7, 2013) 'Marijuana Stops Child's Severe Seizures' http://edition.cnn.com/2013/08/07/health/charlotte-child-medical-marijuana/

[73] Colorado Pot Guide (May 29, 2016) 'Charlotte's Web: The Strain That's Saving Lives' https://www.coloradopotguide.com/colorado-marijuana-blog/article/charlottes-web-the-strain-thats-saving-lives/

[74] Readhead, Harry (August 11, 2015) 'First Legal Charlotte's Web Cannabis Oil to Go on Sale in the UK' http://metro.co.uk/2015/08/11/first-legal-cannabis-oil-to-go-on-sale-in-the-uk-5336811/

[75] The Conversation (March 15, 2016) 'What Is Dravet Syndrome and How Can It Be Managed?' https://theconversation.com/explainer-what-is-dravet-syndrome-and-how-can-it-be-managed-50077

[76] Innes, Emma (August 13, 2013) 'We Feed Our Daughter Cannabis to Stop Her Seizures' http://www.dailymail.co.uk/health/article-2391207/We-feed-daughter-CANNABIS-stop-having-thousands-seizures-week-Parents-say-toddler-say-walk-talk-time-thanks-treatment.html

[77] McClure, James (December 2, 2015) 'Why Florida's Legal Medical Marijuana Strain Is Called Charlotte's Web' https://www.civilized.life/articles/strain-stories-charlottes-web-cannabis/

[78] Gucciardi, Anthony (February 2, 2015) 'Marijuana Backed By More Studies Than Most FDA Approved Drugs.'
http://naturalsociety.com/marijuana-backed-studies-fda-approved-pharma-drugs/

[79] Ferro, Shaunacy (April 18, 2013) 'Why It's So Hard for Scientists to Study Medical Marijuana'
http://www.popsci.com/science/article/2013-04/why-its-so-hard-scientists-study-pot

[80] Zuardi et al. (2008) 'Cannabidiol for the Treatment of Psychosis in Parkinson's Disease' British Association for Psychopharmacology
http://jop.sagepub.com/content/23/8/979

[81] Tartokovsky, Margarita (Retrieved October 14, 2016) 'What You Need to Know about Psychosis in Parkinson's Disease'
http://psychcentral.com/lib/what-you-need-to-know-about-psychosis-in-parkinsons-disease/

[82] Psychiatric Times (April 12, 2013) 'BPRS: Brief Psychiatric Rating Scale' http://www.psychiatrictimes.com/clinical-scales-schizophrenia/clinical-scales-schizophrenia/bprs-brief-psychiatric-rating-scale

[83] Brandstaedter et al. (2005) 'Development and Evaluation of the Parkinson Psychosis Questionnaire' https://www.infona.pl/resource/bwmeta1.element.springer-e21e6a7c-fd15-3c6a-a0ca-6a252faeb953

[84] Granowicz, Julia (May 22, 2016) 'Could Medical Marijuana Benefit Parkinson's Patients?' https://www.marijuanatimes.org/could-medical-marijuana-benefit-parkinsons-disease-patients/

[85] Crippa et al. (2012) 'Cannabidiol for the Treatment of Cannabis Withdrawal Syndrome' http://onlinelibrary.wiley.com/doi/10.1111/jcpt.12018/full

[86] Wilson, Clare (May 6, 2015) 'Withdrawal Drug Could Help Cannabis Addicts Kick the Habit' https://www.newscientist.com/article/mg22630204-500-

withdrawal-drug-could-help-cannabis-addicts-kick-the-habit/

[87] Copeland et al. (2014) 'Cannabidiol for the Management of Cannabis Withdrawal' https://ndarc.med.unsw.edu.au/project/cannabidiol-cbd-management-cannabis-withdrawal-phase-ii-proof-concept-open-label-study#menu_item_6

[88] Ligresti et al. (2006) 'Anti-Tumor Activity of Plant Cannabinoids on Human Breast Carcinoma' The Journal of Pharmacology http://www.medicinalgenomics.com/cannabidiol-dramatically-inhibits-breast-cancer-cell-growth-study-says/

[89] Mandal, Ananya (Retrieved October 13, 2016) 'What Is Autophagy?' http://www.news-medical.net/health/What-is-Autophagy.aspx

[90] Shrivastava et al. (2011) 'Cannabidiol Induces Programmed Cell Death' Molecular Cancer Therapeutics http://mct.aacrjournals.org/content/10/7/1161

[91] Cilio et al. (2014) 'The Case for Assessing Cannabidiol in Epilepsy' Epilepsia http://onlinelibrary.wiley.com/doi/10.1111/epi.12635/full

[92] Devinsky et al. (2016) 'Cannabidiol in Patients with Treatment Resistant Epilepsy' The Lancet http://www.thelancet.com/journals/laneur/article/PIIS1474-4422(15)00379-8/abstract

[93] Leo et al. (2016) 'Cannabidiol and Epilepsy: Rationale and Therapeutic Potential' Pharmacological Research http://www.sciencedirect.com/science/article/pii/S1043661816301797

[94] Aviello et al. (2012) 'Chemopreventive Effect of Cannabidiol on Experimental Colon Cancer' Journal of Molecular Medicine http://link.springer.com/article/10.1007/s00109-011-0856-x

[95] Dorm, Drake (Retrieved 13 October 2016) 'Study Shows Cannabis Extracts May Treat Colon Cancer'

https://www.medicaljane.com/2014/01/09/study-cannabis-extracts-rich-in-cannabidiol-cbd-may-effectively-treat-colon-cancer/

[96] Crippa et al. (2003) 'Effects of Cannabidiol on Regional Cerebral Blood Flow' Neuropsychopharmacology http://www.cannextract.ro/images/uploaded/Neuropsychopharmacology%20-%20Effects%20of%20Cannabidiol%20(CBD)%20on%20Regional%20Cerebral%20Blood%20Flow.pdf

[97] Gofshteyn et al. (2016) 'Cannabidiol as a Potential Treatment for FIRES in the Acute and Chronic Phases' Journal of Child Neurology http://jcn.sagepub.com/content/early/2016/09/20/0883073816669450.abstract

[98] Genetic and Rare Diseases Information Center (Retrieved October 20, 2016) 'Febrile Infection Related Epilepsy Syndrome' https://rarediseases.info.nih.gov/diseases/11005/febrile-infection-related-epilepsy-syndrome

[99] Waltz, Vanessa (January 27, 2014) 'Branden the Brave's Battle for Medical Cannabis Access'

http://www.ladybud.com/2014/01/27/fighting-fires-branden-the-braves-fight-for-medical-cannabis-access/

[100] Englund et al. (2012) 'Cannabidiol Inhibits THC Elicited Paranoid Symptoms and Memory Impairment' Journal of Psychopharmacology http://jop.sagepub.com/content/27/1/19.short

[101] High Times (December 9, 2014). 'The Simple Answer: What Are CBD and THC?' http://hightimes.com/medicinal/science/the-simple-answer-what-are-thc-cbd/

[102] Niesink and Laar (2013) 'Does Cannabidiol Protect Against the Adverse Psychological Effects of THC?' Front Psychology https://www.ncbi.nlm.nih.gov/pmc/articles/PMC3797438/

[103] Kay et al. (Retrieved October 20, 2016) 'Positive and Negative Syndrome Scale' http://www.mhs.com/product.aspx?gr=cli&id=overview&prod=panss

[104] Geffrey et al. (2015) 'Drug-Drug Interaction between Clobazam and Cannabidiol in Children with Refractory Epilepsy' Epilepsia.
http://onlinelibrary.wiley.com/doi/10.1111/epi.13060/full

[105] Drugs (Retrieved October 20, 2016) 'Clobazam.'
https://www.drugs.com/cdi/clobazam.html

[106] Devitt Lee, Adrian (September 8, 2015)' CBD Drug Interactions: Role of Cytochrome P450'
https://www.projectcbd.org/article/cbd-drug-interactions-role-cytochrome-p450

[107] Neurology Reviews (Retrieved October 19, 2016) 'Two Studies Provide Update on Effectiveness of Cannabidiol in Patients with Epilepsy'
http://www.mdedge.com/neurologyreviews/article/89073/epilepsy-seizures/two-studies-provide-update-effectiveness

[108] Avraham et al. (2011) 'Cannabidiol Improves Brain and Liver Function in a Hepatic Failure Induced Model of Encephalopathy in Mice' British Journal of Pharmacology.

http://onlinelibrary.wiley.com/doi/10.1111/j.1476-5381.2010.01179.x/full

[109] NHS (Retrieved October 19, 2016) 'Liver Disease' http://www.nhs.uk/conditions/liver-disease/pages/introduction.aspx

[110] Robel et al. (2015) 'Reactive Astrogliosis Causes the Development of Spontaneous Seizures' The Journal of Neuroscience

[111] Alswat, K (2013) 'The Role of Endocannabinoids System in Fatty Liver Disease and Therapeutic Potentials' http://www.saudijgastro.com/article.asp?issn=1319-3767;year=2013;volume=19;issue=4;spage=144;epage=151;aulast=Alswat

[112] Bergamaschi et al. (2011) 'Cannabidiol Reduces the Anxiety Induced by Simulated Public Speaking in Social Phobia Patients' Neuropharmacology http://www.nature.com/npp/journal/v36/n6/abs/npp20116a.html

[113] Cho, Jeena (June 1, 2016) '13 Things about Social Anxiety Disorder You May Not Have Known' http://www.forbes.com/sites/jeenacho/2016/06/01/13-things-about-social-anxiety-disorder-you-may-not-have-known/#4a4dd57559c2

[114] Social Anxiety (Retrieved October 20, 2016) 'When Fear of Public Speaking is an Anxiety Disorder' http://www.social-anxiety.com/when-fear-of-public-speaking-is-an-anxiety-disorder/

[115] White, Shelley (August 2, 2015) 'Research Shows CBD Combats Social Anxiety' http://www.collective-evolution.com/2015/08/02/research-shows-cbd-combats-social-anxiety/

[116] Killgore (1999) 'Can a Single Item Scale Accurately Classify Depressive Mood State?' Psychological Reports http://prx.sagepub.com/content/85/3_suppl/1238.refs

[117] Brinthaupt et al. (2003) 'The Self Talk Scale: Development, Factor Analysis, and Validation' Journal of

Personality Assessment
http://www.tandfonline.com/doi/abs/10.1080/00223890802484498?src=recsys&journalCode=hjpa20

[118] Giddingson, Jack (November 20, 2013) 'Cannabidiol: The Side of Marijuana You Don't Know'
http://www.chicagonow.com/chicago-medical-marijuana/2013/11/cannabidiol-the-side-of-marijuana-you-dont-know/

[119] Karanicolas et al. (2010) 'Blinding: Who, What, When, Why, How?' PMC
https://www.ncbi.nlm.nih.gov/pmc/articles/PMC2947122/

[120] Liou et al. (2006) 'Neuroprotective and Blood Retinal Barrier Preserving Effects of Cannabidiol in Experimental Diabetes' The American Journal of Pathology.
http://www.sciencedirect.com/science/article/pii/S000294401062086X

[121] American Academy of Ophthalmology (Retrieved October 19) 'What Is Diabetic Retinopathy?'
http://www.aao.org/eye-health/diseases/what-is-diabetic-retinopathy

[122] Best Health (Retrieved October 19, 2016) '5 Health Conditions That Are Caused By Diabetes' http://www.besthealthmag.ca/best-you/diabetes/5-health-conditions-that-are-caused-by-diabetes/

[123] Mayo Clinic (Retrieved October 19, 2016) 'Diabetes Treatment: Using Insulin to Manage Blood Sugar' http://www.mayoclinic.org/diseases-conditions/diabetes/in-depth/diabetes-treatment/art-20044084

[124] Science Daily (February 27, 2006) 'Marijuana Compound May Help Stop Diabetic Retinopathy' https://www.sciencedaily.com/releases/2006/02/060227184647.htm

[125] National Eye Institute (Retrieved October 19, 2016) 'Facts about Diabetic Eye Disease' https://nei.nih.gov/health/diabetic/retinopathy

[126] Modi et al. (2016) 'Cannabidiol Use Leading to Regression of a Pituitary Macroadenoma' Endocrine

Society
http://press.endocrine.org/doi/abs/10.1210/endo-meetings.2016.NP.18.SUN-484

[127] Cancer Research UK (Retrieved October 18, 2016) ‘Cannabis, Cannabinoids, and Cancer: The Evidence So Far’
http://scienceblog.cancerresearchuk.org/2012/07/25/cannabis-cannabinoids-and-cancer-the-evidence-so-far/

[128] John Hopkins Medicine (Retrieved October 19, 2016) ‘Pituitary Tumors’
http://www.hopkinsmedicine.org/healthlibrary/conditions/endocrinology/pituitary_tumors_85,P00424/

[129] Potter, Lewis (Retrieved October 19, 2016) ‘What Is Cushing’s syndrome?’
http://geekymedics.com/cushings-syndrome/

[130] University of Iowa Healthcare (Retrieved October 19, 2016) ‘Pituitary Adenoma Causing Compression of the Optic Chiasm’
http://webeye.ophth.uiowa.edu/eyeforum/cases/177-pituitary-adenoma.htm

[131] Velasco et al. (2016) 'The Use of Cannabinoids as Anticancer Agents' Progress in Neuro-Psychopharmacology and Biological Psychiatry http://www.sciencedirect.com/science/article/pii/S0278584615001190

[132] Gomes et al. (2012) 'Cannabidiol Administration Alters Cardiovascular Responses Induced by Acute Restraint Stress through 5-HT1A Receptor' European Neuropsychopharmacology

https://www.researchgate.net/publication/232220389_Cannabidiol_administration_into_the_bed_nucleus_of_the_stria_terminalis_alters_cardiovascular_responses_induced_by_acute_restraint_stress_through_5-HTA_receptor

[133] Lee et al. (2016) 'Cannabidiol Limits T Cell Mediated Chronic Autoimmune Myocarditis' Europe PMC http://europepmc.org/abstract/med/26772776

[134] Myocarditis Foundation (Retrieved October 20, 2016) ‘Myocarditis Causes, Treatments, Symptoms’ http://www.myocarditisfoundation.org/about-myocarditis/

[135] Nagarkatti et al. (2011) ‘Do Cannabinoids Have a Therapeutic Role in Organ Transplantation?’ PMC https://www.ncbi.nlm.nih.gov/pmc/articles/PMC2923447/

[136] Chemo Care (Retrieved October 20, 2016) ‘Myocarditis’ http://chemocare.com/chemotherapy/side-effects/myocarditis.aspx

[137] Zanelati et al. (2009) ‘Antidepressant Effects of Cannabidiol in Mice’ British Journal of Pharmacology http://onlinelibrary.wiley.com/doi/10.1111/j.1476-5381.2009.00521.x/full

[138] Can et al. (2012) ‘The Mouse Forced Swim Test’ PMC https://www.ncbi.nlm.nih.gov/pmc/articles/PMC3353513/

[139] Slattery and Cryan (2012) 'Using the Rat Forced Swim Test to Assess Antidepressant Activity in Rodents' Nature Protocols http://www.nature.com/nprot/journal/v7/n6/full/nprot.2012.044.html

[140] Franko et al. (2015) 'The Forced Swim Test as a Model of Depressive Like Behaviour' Jove https://www.jove.com/video/52587/the-forced-swim-test-as-a-model-of-depressive-like-behavior

[141] Bekoff, Mark (January 5, 2012) 'Drowning Rats and Human Depression' https://www.psychologytoday.com/blog/animal-emotions/201201/drowning-rats-and-human-depression-positive-psychology-whom

[142] Mind (Retrieved October 20, 2016) 'Antidepressants A-Z' http://www.mind.org.uk/information-support/drugs-and-treatments/antidepressants-a-z/imipramine/

[143] Weiss et al. (2008) 'Cannabidiol Arrests Onset of Autoimmune Diabetes in NOD Mice' Neuropharmacology

http://www.sciencedirect.com/science/article/pii/S0028390807001888

[144] Ketchiff, Mirel (Retrieved October 20, 2016) '7 Silent Symptoms of Pre-Diabetes'
http://www.shape.com/lifestyle/mind-and-body/7-silent-symptoms-pre-diabetes

[145] Sheldrick, Giles (January 28, 2014) 'Diabetes Experts Confident They Can Wipe Out Killer Disease in 25 Years'
http://www.express.co.uk/life-style/health/456505/Diabetes-experts-confident-they-can-wipe-out-killer-disease-in-20-years

[146] Thermofisher Scientific (June 2012) 'When Inflammatory Cytokines are Unbalanced' Bioprobes Journal of Cell Biology
https://www.thermofisher.com/uk/en/home/references/newsletters-and-journals/bioprobes-journal-of-cell-biology-applications/bioprobes-issues-2012/bioprobes-67-june-2012/immunoassays-inflammation-cytokines.html#

[147] Braun and Rorsman (2013) 'Regulation of Insulin Secretion in Human Pancreatic Islets' Annual Review of Physiology http://www.annualreviews.org/doi/abs/10.1146/annurev-physiol-030212-183754?journalCode=physiol

[148] Diabetes (April 24, 2015) 'Compound in Cannabis Could Treat Diabetes' http://www.diabetes.co.uk/news/2015/Apr/cbd-compound-in-cannabis-could-treat-diabetes,-researchers-suggest-95335970.html

[149] Lukehelo and Motadi (2016) 'Cannabidiol Extracts Inhibit Cell Growth and Induce Apoptosis in Cervical Cancer Cells' BMC Complementary and Alternative Medicine https://bmccomplementalternmed.biomedcentral.com/articles/10.1186/s12906-016-1280-0

[150] National Institute of Drug Abuse (July 20, 2016) 'Researching Marijuana for Therapeutic Purposes' https://www.drugabuse.gov/about-nida/noras-blog/2015/07/researching-marijuana-therapeutic-purposes-potential-promise-cannabidiol-cbd

[151] Cure FFI (April 28, 2013) 'Cell Biology 11: Apoptosis and Necrosis' http://www.cureffi.org/2013/04/28/cell-biology-11-apoptosis-necrosis/

[152] NCBI (Retrieved October 20, 2016) 'The P53 Tumor Suppressor Protein' https://www.ncbi.nlm.nih.gov/books/NBK22268/

[153] R&D Systems (Retrieved October 20, 2016) 'Apoptosis: Caspase Pathways' https://www.rndsystems.com/resources/articles/apoptosis-caspase-pathways

[154] Levin, Sam (May 9, 2016) 'Medical Marijuana Draws Parents to US' https://www.theguardian.com/society/2016/may/09/medical-marijuana-families-move-to-colorado-epilepsy

[155] Chesher et al. (2012) 'Interaction of Cannabis and General Anesthetic' British Journal of Pharmacology http://onlinelibrary.wiley.com/doi/10.1111/j.1476-5381.1974.tb08594.x/abstract

[156] Paton and Pertwee (1972) 'Effects of Cannabis and Its Constituents on Pentobarbitone Sleeping Time' NCBI https://www.ncbi.nlm.nih.gov/pubmed/4668592

[157] McGreevey, Sue (July 24, 2009) 'MGH Researchers Develop Potentially Safer General Anesthetic' http://news.harvard.edu/gazette/story/2009/07/mgh-researchers-develop-potentially-safer-general-anesthetic/

[158] Bang, S. (2015) 'How We Manage Our Most Vulnerable Patients' NCBI https://www.ncbi.nlm.nih.gov/pmc/articles/PMC4610921/

[159] Das et al. (2013) 'Cannabidiol Enhances Consolidation of Explicit Fear Extinction in Humans' Psychopharmacology

http://link.springer.com/article/10.1007/s00213-012-2955-y

[160] Mueller and Quirk (2007) 'Neural Mechanisms of Extinction Learning and Retrieval' PMC https://www.ncbi.nlm.nih.gov/pmc/articles/PMC2668714/

[161] Lamia, Mary (December 15, 2011) 'The Complexity of Fear' https://www.psychologytoday.com/blog/intense-emotions-and-strong-feelings/201112/the-complexity-fear

[162] Inglis-Arkell, Esther (March 6, 2011) 'Ten Fear Responses That Make No Sense and Why We Have Them' http://io9.gizmodo.com/5808083/ten-fear-responses-that-make-no-sense-and-why-we-have-them

[163] World Health (June 12, 2014) 'Cannabidiol Confers Anti-Anxiety Effects' http://www.worldhealth.net/news/cannabidiol-confers-anti-anxiety-effects/

[164] Britton et al. (2014) 'Looking Beyond Fear and Extinction Learning' PMC https://www.ncbi.nlm.nih.gov/pmc/articles/PMC4333677/

[165] Silva et al. (2014) Cannabidiol Normalises Protein Expression Levels in Rats with Brain Iron Overload' Molecular Neurobiology http://link.springer.com/article/10.1007/s12035-013-8514-7

[166] Zecca et al. (2004) 'Iron, Brain Aging, and Neurodegenerative Disorders' Nature Reviews Neuroscience http://www.nature.com/nrn/journal/v5/n11/full/nrn1537.html

[167] Mazarakis et al. (1997) 'Apoptosis in Neural Development and Disease' http://fn.bmj.com/content/77/3/F165.full

[168] Adams et al. (2015) 'Architecture of the Synaptophysin/Synaptobrevin Complex' Scientific Reports http://www.nature.com/articles/srep13659

[169] Dorm, Drake (Retrieved October 20, 2016) 'Cannabidiol May Help to Prevent or Treat Neurodegenerative Disease'

https://www.medicaljane.com/2013/08/15/how-cannabidiol-cbd-can-protect-against-neurodegenerative-disease/

[170] FDA (June 24, 2015) 'Cannabidiol: Barriers to Research'
http://www.fda.gov/NewsEvents/Testimony/ucm453989.htm

[171] Roy, Remi (May 3, 2016) 'Leading Scientists Discuss the Future of Cannabis Research'

https://news.lift.co/leading-scientists-discuss-future-cannabis-research/

[172] Quit Smoking Community (Retrieved October 20, 2016) 'A Comprehensive Guide on How to Choose the Best CBD Oil'
https://quitsmokingcommunity.org/best-cbd-oil/

[173] Burnett, Malik (Retrieved October 21, 2016) 'Finding the Optimal Therapeutic Ratio between CBD and THC'

https://www.medicaljane.com/2014/05/29/finding-the-optimal-therapeutic-ratio-of-thc-and-cbd/

[174] Life Enthusiast (May 16, 2015) 'Hemp Oil is Changing Chronic Pain Management' http://www.life-enthusiast.com/health-news/hemp-oil-is-changing-chronic-pain-management/

[175] Henein, Mariam (August 10, 2016) 'What to Look For When Buying CBD Medical Hemp Oil' https://www.honeycolony.com/article/4-things-to-look-for-when-buying-cbd-medical-hemp-oil/

[176] Health Canada (Retrieved October 20, 2016) 'About Hemp and Canada's Hemp Industry' http://www.hc-sc.gc.ca/hc-ps/substancontrol/hemp-chanvre/about-apropos/faq/index-eng.php

[177] Health Table (April 11, 2016) '7 Things to Consider When Buying Hemp Seeds' http://www.healthable.org/7-things-to-consider-when-buying-hemp-seeds/

[178] Eckelkamp, Stephanie (January 14, 2015) 'The 6 Healthiest Protein Powders for Your Smoothie' http://www.prevention.com/food/healthy-eating-tips/best-protein-powders-for-smoothies

[179] Shortsleeve, Cassie (Retrieved October 21, 2016) 'What Is the Best Vegan Protein Powder?' http://www.mensfitness.com/nutrition/supplements/whats-best-vegan-protein-powder

49350809R00093

Made in the USA
Columbia, SC
20 January 2019